# Bridging Medicine and Miracles

By

Susan Jeffrey Busen

# Bridging Medicine and Miracles

Essential Truths, Key Practices, and a New Perspective on Health and Healing



Note to the Reader

The information, ideas, and suggestions presented in this book are not intended as a substitute for professional advice. Before following any suggestions contained in this book, you should consult your personal physician or mental health professional. Emotional Freedom Techniques and the GetSet™ Approach are considered experimental procedures. You must take complete responsibility for your decision to act based on any suggestions presented herein. Neither the author nor the publisher shall be liable or responsible for any loss or damage allegedly arising as a consequence of your use or application of any information or suggestions in this book. The information and suggestions in this book are not intended to diagnose, treat, cure, heal, or prevent any mental or physical condition. If you think you have a medical condition, consult a licensed medical professional.

Visit www.TapintoBalance.com to claim your free downloadable gift.

ISBN-10: 0-9820697-5-8

ISBN-13: 978-0-9820697-5-2

Printed in the United States of America

# Dedication

For Lily

## Also by Susan Jeffrey Busen

*Tap into Joy: A Guide to Emotional Freedom Techniques for Kids and Their Parents*
*Tap into Success: A Guide to Thriving in College Using Emotional Freedom Techniques*
*Tap into Balance: Your Guide to Awakening the Joy Within Using the GetSet™ Approach*
*Good Vibes: 48 Tips to Raise YOUR Vibration—The Secret to Creating a Healthy Lifestyle and Attracting What You Want*
*Tap into Joy: Energy Clearing for Children of All Ages* DVD
EFT タッピングセラピー おとなが子どもにできること
(*Tap into Joy* in Japanese)

Upcoming Books:

*Tormented by Technology: How to Protect Yourself from an Impending Crisis*
*Tap into Your Dream: The Secret to Creating the Life You Want*
*Tap into Hope: A Guide to Helping Children through Grief*
Coauthor of *Outside In: A Guided Journal of Self-Reflection and Awakening*
*Tap into Joy* in Korean

Contributing Author:

*Cancer: From Tears to Triumph*
*My Creative Thoughts Journal*
*My Big Idea Book*

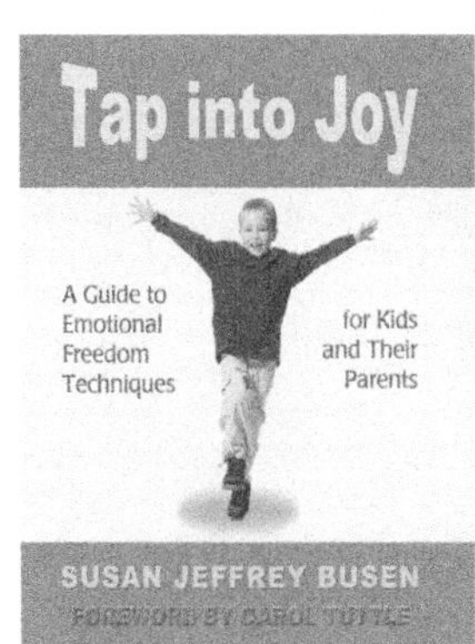
Tap into Joy
A Guide to Emotional Freedom Techniques
for Kids and Their Parents
SUSAN JEFFREY BUSEN

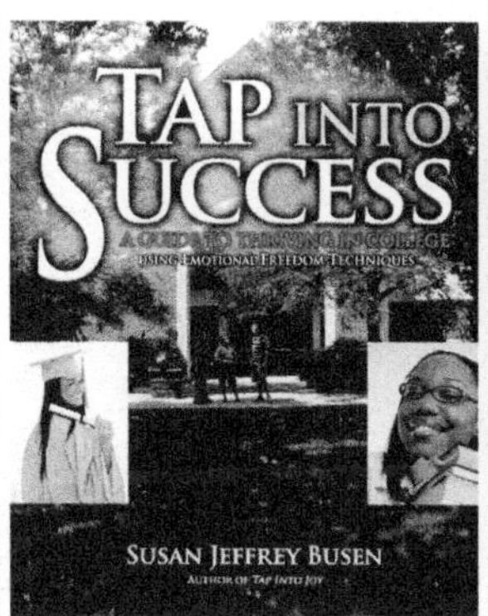
TAP INTO SUCCESS
USING EMOTIONAL FREEDOM TECHNIQUES
SUSAN JEFFREY BUSEN

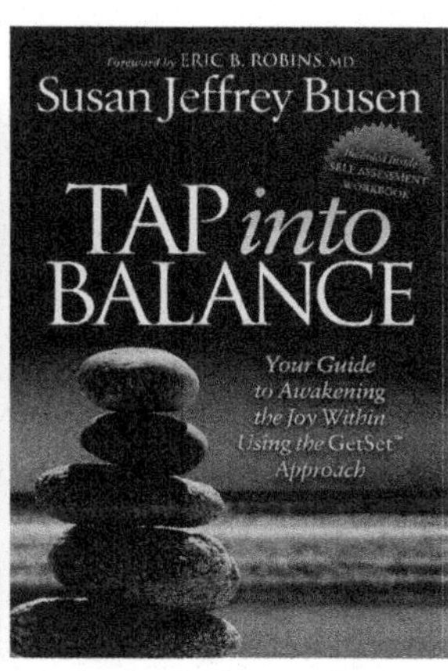
Foreword by ERIC B. ROBINS, MD
Susan Jeffrey Busen
TAP into BALANCE
Your Guide to Awakening the Joy Within Using the GetSet™ Approach

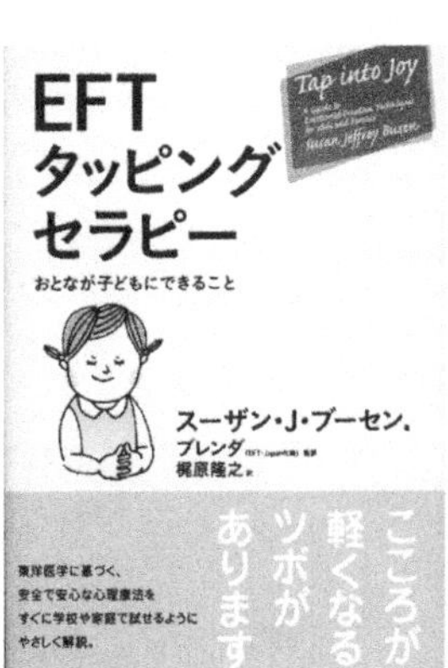
EFT
タッピングセラピー
おとなが子どもにできること
スーザン・J・ブーセン。
こころが軽くなるツボがあります。

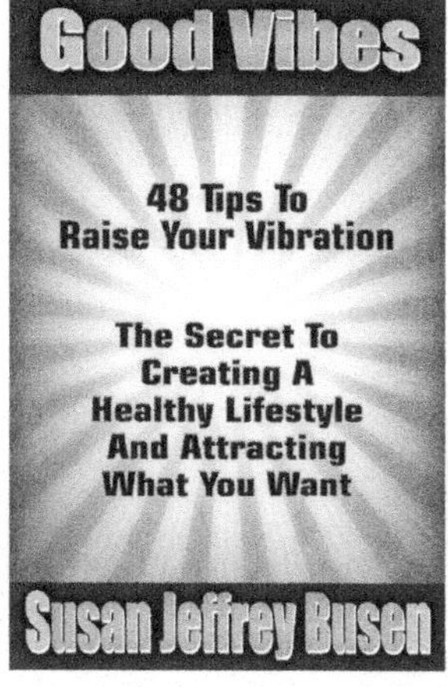
Good Vibes
48 Tips To Raise Your Vibration
The Secret To Creating A Healthy Lifestyle And Attracting What You Want
Susan Jeffrey Busen

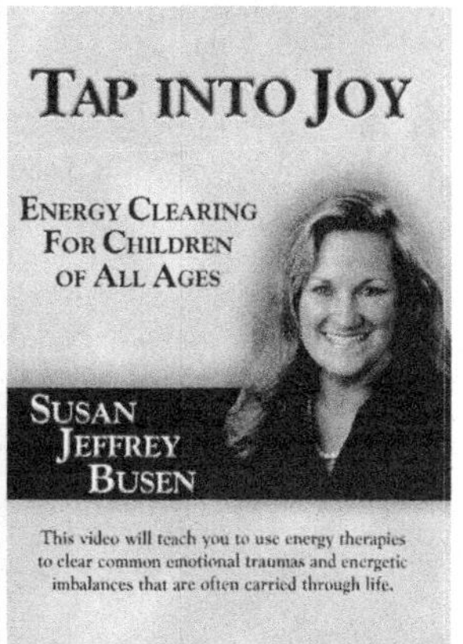
TAP INTO JOY
ENERGY CLEARING FOR CHILDREN OF ALL AGES
SUSAN JEFFREY BUSEN
This video will teach you to use energy therapies to clear common emotional traumas and energetic imbalances that are often carried through life.

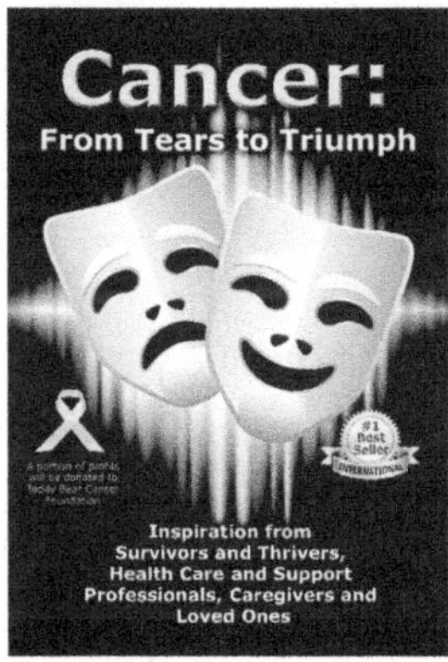
Cancer:
From Tears to Triumph
Inspiration from Survivors and Thrivers, Health Care and Support Professionals, Caregivers and Loved Ones

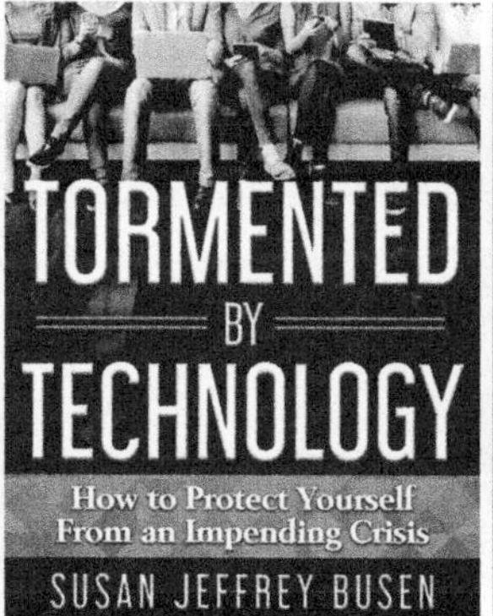
TORMENTED BY TECHNOLOGY
How to Protect Yourself From an Impending Crisis
SUSAN JEFFREY BUSEN

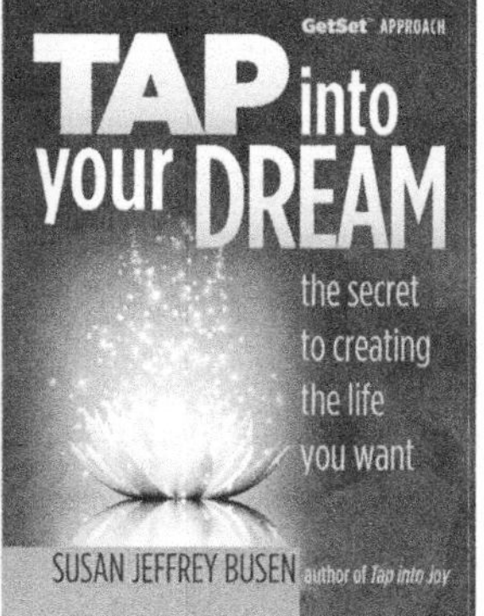
GetSet™ APPROACH
TAP into your DREAM
the secret to creating the life you want
SUSAN JEFFREY BUSEN author of Tap into Joy

# Table of Contents

# Acknowledgments

I am deeply grateful to the following:

My three sons, "The Busen Bros": Tom, Will, and Dan. I don't think I could be more proud of the young men you have become. I am so very honored to be your mom. You inspire me to do my work in the world. I am blessed by your unwavering encouragement.

To Lisa LaJoie for having the courage and wisdom to bring forth a message that encouraged me to write this book even before life presented all the topics.

To Justin Spizman for your guidance in conceptualizing this book, your patience and willingness to work around the obstacles I faced, your brilliant suggestions, and your meticulous attention to detail in editing.

To Lu Jeffrey, Tom Busen, Angie Kiesling, and Cheryl Ross for your editing guidance and the time you devoted to making this a better book.

To Viki Winterton for your generous spirit and help in launching this work.

To all of my family, friends, and medical team who have stuck by me through the devastating illness of electromagnetic hypersensitivity (EHS), who supported and honored my decisions, listened, held space for me as I figured out what was going on and how to begin my healing journey, for helping to reduce your radiation when we are together, for helping me in some way, for inspiring me, or for encouraging me to write or stay accountable with this book, especially: Dan Busen, Tom Busen, Will Busen, Karen Jeffrey, Lu Jeffrey, Dr. Alex Bennet, Dr. Birhanu, Jack Canfield, Jake Huff, Jo Ann Huff, Michelle Lopez, Don Nowaczyk, Hal Price, Brandon Puk, Michelle Sanford, John Sterling, and Marcia Wieder.

To Jeffrey Smith, mentor and fellow non-GMO activist, thank you for your dedication to this cause, leading this movement, and for teaching me to speak out and educate others.

To Dietrich Klinghardt, MD, PhD, for your courage and work in the health effects of electromagnetic radiation.

To some of my favorite guys who support me from the other side: my dad, Tom Jeffrey, my brother, Tom Jeffrey, and Hank Loukota. Also, to Richard Fammeree, who inspired me to always look within, and to Jim Walters, who always inspired me to think outside the box.

Thank you to everyone who has purchased this book and for trusting me to be a part of your journey. I am truly honored. May this book empower you with the knowledge and tools you need to thrive.

# Preface

In *Bridging Medicine and Miracles*, I offer you perspective and thoughts about health and healing. I am not trying to influence you on any particular form of treatment, but rather educate you as to all options and alternatives available. I am sharing my opinions and beliefs based on my own story, my years of work in toxicology, in government and corporate research, a lifetime of my own health challenges, my experience working with thousands of clients over nearly two decades to help them discover and implement healing in their own lives, my experiences with medicine, working in the medical field, and studying holistic modalities.

I am writing to people who desire a higher level of health and want to live to the best of their ability, for those young adults who are just beginning to take charge of and be proactive about their health, and for those in any age group who may be experiencing a health challenge or mystery symptoms that traditional medicine cannot explain. I am writing to those who are looking for answers and a better way to take care of themselves.

I'll share what I've discovered throughout the course of my life about how you can overcome the challenges in your life. I have devoted decades to researching topics related to health and healing, toxins, and dis-ease, and offer my opinions on each of these relevant subjects. As you navigate through this book, ask yourself how this information might help you adopt healthy practices, evolve, and even heal.

I may be challenging your belief systems. You may not believe everything you read in this book. Take what resonates with you because that will be most useful in your healing and well-being. My intention is not to discredit any field or industry, but to point out areas they may be falling short in, to let you know that you do have options, and to invite you to take the information I present and to make the choices that feel best to you. Knowledge is power. You may not feel comfortable seeking holistic care. Traditional medicine may be your answer. I have tremendous respect for the medical field, and I stay connected so I can best serve from both perspectives. There is no right answer, only careful consideration of the options in front of you.

I have often been asked how I do what I do. First, let me be clear that I am not a doctor or therapist. I am not licensed to practice any form of medicine. While I help facilitate, investigate, and educate, the healing does not come from me. I have assisted many people to physically, emotionally, or spiritually heal something in their life. It is about giving them information and empowering them to take action toward healing. We are all healers, but most of us have not yet realized this.

I have spent time with many clients over the years in my coaching practice and with patients in the medical field. One of my learned gifts is that of being able to hear people. I don't mean simply listen. I hear them, I hear their pain, I listen to their story, and I feel them. This level of empathy has given me the ability to be quite effective in what I do.

When working with a client, my intention is to help that person get relief, freedom from his or her symptoms, clarity, and healing. I expect that this will happen. I have unshakeable confidence that all the pieces I can bring to the table are in place. I have no control over what my clients bring and what they will do with the insights that I present to them. When clients ask if I can help them, I say that I'd like to. I really don't know. I work to determine the causes and imbalances within their bodies and minds to restore balance. It is often based on my gut instincts and intuition. I work with newborns through people at the end of life and with animals. What I find most intriguing about this is that many of my clients come to me after many years of seeking specialty medical help or even decades of counseling without the level of success they would like. Sometimes, I am their last hope. Many admit that they don't know what else to do, but they are hungry for answers and results. I believe that hunger is responsible for a big part of their success. The truth is I am just providing them with insights and direction. When they make up their mind to heal and put the pieces in place, with whatever information or treatments they choose to use, they heal. I encourage you to have an insatiable appetite for the answers that you need. Never resign yourself to circumstances if you are not happy with them.

I believe all healing comes from a higher source. I call that source God or the divine, the Holy Spirit, the Creator, the universe, your higher power, universal love, Buddha, or Source. You may call it something else. We diminish its power and expansiveness simply by putting a name on it. We all worship in our own way. I honor your belief, whatever it may be. There is a mystical or spiritual force that cannot be denied. I believe it has been in existence long before any organized religions. It is the divine intelligence of all life. It cannot be seen in a concrete manner or scientifically measured. We simply believe it exists and surrender to it.

I believe all dis-ease has one thing in common—a lack of health and balance. I have devoted a large portion of my life to learning how to identify the causes of disease in order to help people find solutions. I have been given a gift to feel and move energy. I have always had a highly developed sense of intuition. Since I was a young child I knew things and experienced things that others didn't quite understand. I thought everyone had these insights and abilities. The awareness that others didn't understand intuition, didn't believe in it, or thought it was somehow bad made me uncomfortable. It scared me. For a long time I hid it and hoped it would go away. Now I embrace and appreciate this ability. I have come to realize that everyone has it even if they haven't learned to trust it.

Some may label me, my opinions, or methods as quackery. I urge you not to judge it because, when you are facing a crisis, it may be the very thing that saves your life. When we think outside the box we are sometimes considered New Age. That is a scary term for many because they don't always understand it. Some even label it as some dark, cultlike belief system. These fears limit our thinking and our ability to seek the answers we may need. From my perspective, it could not be further from the truth. It is based on sensible, objective thinking. Do not take any action that is not in alignment with your spiritual beliefs.

There will be people who will dispute what I say and discredit me for what I have written in this book. Be aware that there are industries and organizations that pay people to discredit those who bring forth truths that may harm their financial or business interests. My motive is only to share my experiences in a way that will help others. I do not intend to convince anyone of my viewpoints or judge others for theirs. I am simply providing the information, giving you some ideas on how you can reduce your exposure to things that may be harming you, and leaving the rest up to you. I believe it is my purpose to expose these things and give my opinion at any cost. I know the cost of not doing it. If I did not fulfill my purpose and answer the call, I would be doing a disservice to humanity and wasting my time here on the planet. Use the information in this book in a way that feels right to you.

There is turmoil and conflict in the world. We can feed it or we can change it. Humanity is healing. The world needs enlightened people now more than ever. As you gain awareness you realize the power you have to create your life the way you want it. We are all here to learn, explore, and grow; to discover the truth of who we are. I have as much work to do on myself as anyone else. We are all works in progress. Each step we take toward becoming more of our true self puts us in alignment with our purpose. When we feel better, we do better, and we can do more with our life. It is my deepest wish that I can help you find a missing component that will contribute to your health and well-being. Expect miracles. They are everywhere!

# Section I

## The Body and the Importance of Making Informed Choices

You have a tremendous opportunity to experience vibrant health. In fact, your body is designed to heal itself. The chapters in this section are intended to educate and empower you so you can make choices that support your health.

We will explore how our dependence on the medical system is ultimately failing us. We will also discuss and investigate the impact of technology on our bodies, how our reliance on drugs to manage disease has consequences, how food ingredients harm our health, and how we can reduce our environmental impact so we can live in a healthier world.

# Chapter 1

# Introduction

Do you crave more passion and joy? Does the thought of vibrant health excite you? Would you rather spend your seventy-fifth birthday dancing on a cruise ship or confined to a nursing home? Do you want to see your children live a healthy, fulfilling life? Or are you content to see them sitting on the couch watching television while eating frozen dinners? We all have options in front of us. The choices we make for ourselves and our children either support a lifestyle of health and vibrancy or of indifference and disease. It may feel comfortable to sit around and not worry about taking care of ourselves, but is that a meaningful experience of life? Are we willing to risk the long-term consequences?

We all want to get the most out of life and to feel like we are living with purpose and creativity. We want to truly feel alive. The concept of healing has remained a mysterious, uncommon idea for most of us. Yet healing is a continuous process in our bodies, as they have the ability to repair themselves at a cellular level. In addition, we invoke or inhibit healing with our thoughts and beliefs. The ability to heal is at the core of our existence because life wants to support itself. Healing manifests through love and is limited only by our minds. We have more power to heal than we realize.

We are living in very exciting times where we have the best of everything readily available to us. We have good food, modalities that support us at a spiritual level, advanced medical care, technology that we couldn't have imagined five years ago, and simple ways to connect with likeminded people. It is easier than ever to live the life of your dreams. A large segment of society is moving toward more conscious living.

This book is not for those who are content living a life of convenience with no concern for their long-term well-being beyond a hope that it all turns out good. This book is for those who want to be proactive about their health and want to make the best, most informed choices they can to live the best life possible.

If you are a parent, don't you want to feed your kids' bodies and minds healthfully? We have the opportunity to feed our families healthy food in today's fast-paced world. We no longer have to choose quality over price. We have many choices, and it all boils down to understanding your options and making the choices that are most comfortable for you.

Everyone wants to be healthy and happy. While there are some things that only traditional medicine can heal, traditional practices are failing us in preventing disease and maintaining a higher quality of life. We are quickly learning that we need to be proactive and implement a holistic approach to our health. The goal is to use a holistic approach to stay healthy so we don't require medical treatment. I will share my journey and why I believe bridging the two disciplines and finding the balance that works for you is most important.

Lifestyle matters more now than at any time in history. What worked for us a few years ago is no longer working. The status quo is not serving us in the way that we want to live. A few decades ago our food, water, and air were less contaminated than they are today. We had a movement toward convenience. Food scientists enabled us to get our food faster than ever. In fact, we could have some of our food look and feel better, grow with a resistance to certain pesticides, and last longer. All of this was done at a cost.

Now, our air is polluted. Our food is ridden with toxins. Our water is contaminated. Our minds are being continuously fed with negative images. Our bodies are bombarded with radiation. While it is impossible to escape, you can take action to protect yourself from these threats. The choices you make now for yourself and your children have a bigger impact on your health than ever before.

While the health of our planet is declining and the integrity of our food supply is compromised, it is easier than ever to educate ourselves and make informed and less expensive choices. With more people getting on board with healthy lifestyles, we are having a major impact on industries around the world.

Just a few years ago, most people couldn't afford organic food. Ten years ago I was driving thirteen miles to a grocery store to get it. Organic food was difficult to find in grocery stores and on menus. Today, we find it at reasonable prices in major box stores. Most neighborhood grocery stores carry at least some organic, non-GMO, and gluten-free food. We no longer have to go to a fine specialty restaurant to find organic, gluten-free, vegetarian, or vegan options on the menu. Often the corner pizza parlor and local cafes carry a variety of options. Healthy food is now affordable and readily available.

As we get older, we generally become more concerned about our health. But even then, many of us wait until after the system is breaking down to fix it. There is a mindset that many feel they should do what they want, eat what they want, and fix it all later with a magic pill or surgery. The odds are against us if we roll the dice with our health. Regardless of your age and health status, now is the time to be proactive. It is time to honor our bodies and listen to what they are telling us.

When we make poor food choices, we find ourselves feeling bloated, lethargic, mentally foggy, or experiencing any host of other negative symptoms. I call this a food hangover. It's no longer acceptable or worth it. Our bodies recover when we do this on occasion, but it can lead to degenerative problems and disease if it becomes a habit. As I refer to disease or dis-ease throughout this book, I am not only referring to a specific diagnosis or illness but rather any state of disharmony or disruption in the body, in your health, mind, or heart.

We either focus on making our health a priority or we don't. Disease does not happen overnight. It is not our doctor's responsibility to keep us healthy. It is ours. Our habits, behaviors, and choices either harm or support us. The choice is ours, and the divide is more obvious now than ever. I attended a few rock concerts recently where the audience members were predominantly from fifty to seventy years old. It was obvious which people had taken care of themselves and which hadn't.

We feel good when we make good choices. It is empowering to wake up with energy, feeling vibrant and passionate about life. When you have your health, you have your wealth. There is nothing more liberating than to feel good. Just think about the last time you were sick or had a cold. You feel miserable, you can't breathe, you can't sleep, you ache, you have no energy, and everything seems to take tremendous effort. You think back a couple of days and say, "Why can't I feel like that?" or "How much longer until I feel good again?" You feel a bit assaulted by some little microscopic "bug" that has taken away your vitality for a few days.

It takes a little effort, some educating, and a lot of willpower and courage to assess your current lifestyle and change the things that are no longer serving you. The ability to access information and tools to help you and the ability to make healthy choices has never been easier.

Good health is not as elusive as many of us think. We are reinventing how we experience life. It is quite possible that you can enhance your health and quality of life by making gradual changes as outlined in the coming chapters. My intention is to elevate you to a position of empowerment and responsibility.

Some of the ways we are treating problems is no longer serving us. We have to ask ourselves if some of our treatments are making us sicker. Society is more dependent on medication than ever before. I see patients come in with a shopping bag full of prescription drugs. They are taking drugs to manage the side effects of other drugs, not knowing why they are taking some of the drugs they are taking, and they have different doctors prescribing multiple drugs. In some cases, these medications are causing a huge disconnect. They are causing collateral damage and a breakdown in the system. Many are developing addictions to pain medications. Many of the pills that came on the market to help us are harming us. Many of us are tired of seeing illness managed instead of cured.

As a society, we are conditioned to believe traditional medicine is the only way. The truth is that the norm is no longer serving us. Some of the ways we treat problems are not improving our health. Other paradigms merit consideration. We put up barriers to alternative medicine.

However, the truth is that it offers incredibly innovative modalities and mindsets that can enhance our lives on many levels. Humanity craves options. We are living in a very exciting time. Never before have we had so many options and access to food and experiences to keep us healthy. "Alternative" is becoming the norm.

Traditional medicine is necessary in an emergency, for symptoms indicating a serious problem, and for any acute problem that causes you distress. The information I share is intended to supplement, not replace, the advice of your doctor. If you are not getting results when you clean up your diet and lifestyle, you should consult a trusted practitioner or doctor who is open to integration to help you identify the causes. Trust your instincts. If you implement a holistic lifestyle, you may be able to avoid the pills, surgeries, and medical interventions that come with a health crisis. Traditional medicine and alternative medicine are different and should be used differently. Knowing how and when to use both is key to a successful integrative approach to well-being.

This book is not intended to prove that one school of thought is better than the other. It's about educating you, bridging the gap, finding the balance between the two that works best, and helping you create the best life for you and your family.

I have had the privilege of working with and learning from many brilliant doctors and practitioners and have had the honor of helping many clients uncover the causes of their health challenges over the years. Throughout this book, I share stories of my journey that led me to understand how and why our health breaks down and how and why our bodies heal. I share what I did and how I did it in the mind, body, and spirit. I will present what I have learned about both the problems and the possibilities. I spent the first thirty years of my life preparing for a path that I had no idea I was going to take. In this book, I expose what I have learned along the journey.

**We Are Changing the World**

Many of us grew up at a time when much of our food was organic and natural. It did not have to pass inspection or be certified or labeled as such. That was the norm. Today, we think fruit and vegetables are the healthiest food options but they are often the most pesticide-ridden things we eat. Some people view those of us who eat organic food as food snobs who are throwing away money at this “new” food revolution. The truth is that the “cleaner” your food is, the safer it is, the better it tastes, the easier it is for your body to digest, the more filling it is, and the more nutritious it is.

You vote with your dollar. You support these practices whether you know what is going on in the industry or not. You have a moral obligation to support the practices you believe in. You can’t depend on someone else or have blind faith in any institution to oversee the integrity of the product. Agencies and practices are in place to protect you from acute contamination, but they do very little to protect you from the toxic effects from long-term chronic exposure.

When we become educated and avoid purchasing food or products that we believe are not in alignment with our highest interest, we impact the market for that product. I have recently seen an impact from those of us avoiding genetically modified organisms (GMOs), food dyes, and preservatives. We are reaching a tipping point of consumer rejection that is getting the attention of the food industry.

The way to create true change is to boycott the products that are not in alignment with your values and spend your money on those things with which you are in alignment. This gets the attention of corporations and is the best way to shift market practices. When manufacturers see trends in the market, they respond. This makes it progressively easier to identify and purchase healthier food. It is exciting that we are creating these changes as we walk toward healthier, more conscious living.

## My Three Health Crises and Paradigm Shift

In 1992, shortly after having my first baby, I was diagnosed with lupus. The doctor told me that fifteen years was the maximum life expectancy from the time of diagnosis. As I held my newborn baby, I felt fear and anxiety. I had to face the realization that I might not be around to see him through high school. It was terrifying. The more I learned about the disease, the more I dreaded its progression. It forced me to reflect and to question many things. I decided that this was not going to be my fate. It was one of my greatest lessons and an important turning point in my view of disease and of being a victim of my circumstances. At the time, I didn't even realize what I was doing, but this shift in mindset would change the course of my life forever.

Eight years later, I was diagnosed with liver tumors. I found myself in my thirties with three small children facing the reality that my lifestyle was hurting me. I was going for MRIs every six weeks, each time finding more problems. Each MRI showed another cyst, tumor, lesion, or shadow that had to be further investigated. I was being the perfect patient and doing everything the doctor ordered. I came to realize that traditional medicine was failing me. My body was warning me that something I was doing was causing these problems. I was being told to take toxic medications to cover up the symptoms that my body was creating to warn me of impending trouble. Every treatment was causing more dis-ease in my body. It didn't make sense to me. One of my specialists at the time told me the tumors were probably the result of taking over-the-counter pain medications for ten years. My body was toxic, and my liver was overburdened. I didn't think of the tumors as a defect in my body. I knew if I continued on the same path, I could not expect a different result. I was scared, yet I knew there had to be a way to fix this. I did not want to settle for the diagnosis I was given. I felt I had exhausted my options for help healing this with traditional medicine. This was a moment of tremendous power.

I released my inner research scientist and fervently searched for alternatives to fix my health problems. I studied numerous modalities and read all I could about energy, quantum physics, electro-acupuncture, and herbs and homeopathy. As a research scientist, it was a huge paradigm shift to go out on a limb and study alternative modalities. I knew I needed to be open to expand my perspective. I had to consider the possibility that everything I had learned and believed to be true about health and healing might have been an illusion in the first place. I was conditioned to believe in things that did not necessarily serve my body at the highest level. My confusion turned to clarity.

I went into this investigative research to explore alternative medicine with a great deal of discernment and even skepticism. I was a scientist trained and conditioned by the system. At a very core level, I knew there had to be a better way, and as I explored, questioned, and healed, I knew I was on the right path. I began my journey back to health. After a few weeks of being on a self-prescribed protocol, I went for the follow-up MRI to monitor the lesions, cysts, and tumors on my liver.

My physician called to give me the results of the MRI. When I heard his voice I was overcome with weakness, began to sweat, and felt nauseated. Generally a nurse will call with good results, and in that moment I was preparing myself for a grim prognosis. He told me my liver was unremarkable. I asked him to explain, and he said there were no tumors, cysts, or lesions. I was elated that my liver had improved, but quite frankly, I was shocked. I got so excited and was rambling off the things that I was doing. I told him I had been using an energy-related technique and was taking herbs and homeopathics to detoxify and support my liver.

He said, "You can believe whatever you want, but that had nothing to do with it." I was stunned. I can still hear his voice as plain as day. I asked, "What?" Then he repeated his response word for word. My heart sank. I was mortified by his words. I asked, "Scientist to scientist, you don't want to know what I did and why this healed?" I was certain he would want to know how the tumors and cysts disappeared within five weeks. I felt I had stumbled onto a major breakthrough that would advance medicine. I thought he might learn something from my case and be excited that he would have some new ideas to help his other patients. He made it clear that he did not want any further details from me. He didn't even give me a standard response that he would look into it. That was in the early 2000s, and I never returned. Looking back, this was one of the best things that ever happened to me because his blatant disregard for wanting any details fueled an even fiercer curiosity in me.

I wanted to know why he didn't care to hear me out. I wanted to understand why I had developed the tumors while I was doing everything my doctors advised. I wanted to know why traditional medicine was so reluctant to embrace any holistic or alternative ideas on health. I began to question and investigate everything. Most of my initial research was done before I had access to the Internet. Most of it involved ordering books from my local library and traveling around the country to learn different modalities and to meet the right people.

My third health crisis came in 2006, when I was reducing my toxic load by having my dental amalgams replaced with nonmercury fillings. I was not having any problems with my teeth. I had simply concluded that I wanted the mercury out of my body. Shortly after, I began experiencing chronic pain in my jaw and on the right side of my face. I thought it was from the dental work. So naturally, I returned to the dentist. Nothing he did helped fix the problem. I went to a second dentist for another opinion. She wanted to perform root canals on all the teeth in the vicinity of the pain. I did not feel it was the right thing to do.

The pain intensified to the extent that I could not stand it over a period of six months. The only thing I could figure out was that it got worse when my teeth hit together, when I talked or chewed, when I had dental X-rays, when I went through airport scanners, and when I talked on my cell phone. It made no sense to the dentists or me. I tried wearing a mouth guard. I had the dentist grind down all my teeth on the right side of my mouth so they couldn't inadvertently touch each other. Still, I experienced a stabbing pain that came and went in waves. I saw my medical doctor, who could not explain what was causing the pain. It was unbearable. To hide the intense pain from my family, I would go into the basement, walk in circles, hold my face, and cry. I was desperate for answers. No one I turned to was able to help.

One day I had an epiphany. I remembered a client who told me she had a condition she referred to as "the suicide disease." I only knew it caused intense nerve pain and caused her to lock herself in her bedroom for days at a time. I called her. She described the disease, trigeminal neuralgia. I had chills as I listened to her. It felt like she was describing my life.

I did some research on trigeminal neuralgia and found that it is an intermittent misfiring of a cranial nerve that runs from the brain stem and branches out across the face to cause intense stabbing pain. I took my hypothesis to my doctor. He prescribed antiseizure medicine to definitively diagnose the condition. Over several months, I grew dependent on that medication because I didn't know any other way to keep the pain at bay. It had many unpleasant side effects, and I required more and more of it to get through the day. Eventually, I was up to eight pills per day, which caused dizziness, double vision, and weight gain.

Those side effects were not conducive to my busy life as a mother of three active boys. All of my efforts were going into managing the pain and working around the side effects of the medication. I decided there had to be a better way. I was desperate for something to help.

While at a conference, I experienced a mild strain of my wrist. A friend told me about an infrared light that works to reduce pain in achy joints. I felt compelled to learn more and was hopeful that it would relieve the pain in my face. I ordered the light with very high expectations that it would be the answer I needed. I didn't have any other ideas, so I was counting on this being the solution I was longing for. I was in excruciating pain when I got the light, and as I used it, the pain subsided within three minutes. I stopped the medication and have managed the condition without severe pain for about twelve years simply by using the light.

Looking back over that twenty-five-year period, there were a number of similarities in how I overcame those crises that taught me valuable lessons about healing. In all three cases, I went to my doctors and specialists for treatment. I expected them to identify and fix the problem. In each case they either had nothing to offer me or my body did not respond well to the standard treatment.

I now realize that because I believed these conditions would not be my fate and I refused to accept or settle for the diagnosis or treatment I was offered, all of my actions were paving the road and went into alignment with find a better way. I did not know what that way would be and I had never even heard of any of the remedies I used to manage or heal from lupus, liver tumors, and trigeminal neuralgia. I simply knew something better was out there. I believed it, and so it came to be. I attracted what I needed to heal. It was not that I was being naïve to the fact that I had some health challenges that needed to be addressed. Each of them got my attention in a big way. I chose to look at them as warning signs that something was going wrong in my body and I needed to figure out how to either give my body something that it was lacking or take away something that was harming it.

My hope is to help the world expand by opening up a discussion on healing and being a bridge from one school of thought to another and from one belief system to another. I do not proclaim to have all the answers. To find my way, I have combined my knowledge and skills as a research scientist with the perfect mix of health challenges. Along the journey, I struggled with many fears and doubts. I have learned to surrender and trust the process of life.

When I look back over my life, I realize that each trauma, hurt, and disaster unfolded so perfectly that I couldn't have even made up such a magnificent story. In the end, we will all see how perfectly our lives unfolded. We will come to appreciate how much we grew from the challenges we faced and see the miracles we experienced.

## The Perfect Storm

There was a time when I became frustrated with allopathic medicine. I had not yet taken full responsibility for the choices I was making in life, but I realized that the treatment provided by my doctors was seriously harming me. The truth is that I completely shut myself off from traditional medical treatments after my three health challenges. I carried resentment toward the system. I focused on the flaws and lost sight of the benefits. As fate would have it, life was about to teach me a tough lesson.

Shortly after my husband and I separated in 2011, I received a phone call from a local trauma center hospital. The man on the other end of the phone identified himself as a police officer. If you have ever answered a call like that, you know that your life is about to be turned upside down. He told me my husband had been involved in a motorcycle accident. He had serious injuries, and by the time I got to the hospital and the test results came in, the trauma surgeon informed me that he had only minutes to get into surgery or he would not survive. The surgeon said, "Let's go!" and I ran with him and the medical team down the corridor to the operating room. It felt like a scene from a movie.

As we ran, the surgeon explained what was going on, what he needed to do, and asked for my consent. I felt powerless. There was no supplement, homeopathic, or lifestyle change I could recommend that could save my husband. Giving that consent went against everything I believed. It would expose him to lots of radiation, surgery, pathogens, and countless drugs; but I knew it was the only option. As much as I didn't like it, I surrendered.

I sat in the waiting room contemplating the situation, the meaning of life, my purpose, and the purpose of all this as it related to me. I was completely dependent on the medical system and their expertise. I was trying to make sense of it all. At that point, my husband needed surgery and all those machines and drugs to keep him alive.

I spent the next twenty-seven days camped out in the intensive care unit as he remained in a coma with all systems failing. During that time, I got to know the medical team, the life support equipment, the drugs, and the other patients and their families that came and went. I got to know several of the nurses and saw their passion and dedication. I gained an appreciation for each of them. I began to appreciate the machines, the tubes, the tests, and even the drugs. I was intrigued that they could take a body that was near death and keep it functioning until the body could function on its own. As a research scientist and someone with an analytical mind, I wanted to know more. I wanted to understand it.

I began to study each machine that kept him alive. I evaluated the monitors more closely than anyone else. I questioned the nurses and his team until I understood what everything did and what all the numbers meant. I learned to identify each number that was out of range, and I knew what they would need to do to stabilize him. In that highest level of trauma care, lights are never turned off. You lose track of days and survive in a fog. I made trips home each day to pick up the kids and take them where they needed to be. One thing is for certain, if you would have asked me a month prior if I could ever have imagined myself completely dependent on the medical system, I would have said no. Yet at this time I found myself completely dependent on and indebted to it.

Years prior to this incident, I had identified that my husband was sensitive to soybeans. It was not a diagnosed allergic reaction, but he responded negatively and often felt run-down after consuming soy. After the first few days in the coma, medical staff inserted a feeding tube. I read the ingredient list and noticed that the first ingredient was soy. I told the nurse about his sensitivity, and she sort of dismissed it. I told each doctor, and they all sort of believed that he was better off with the "food" than without it. They said since he didn't have an actual allergic reaction and did not break out in hives or experience swelling in the throat or anything drastic, that the benefit of the nutrients outweighed the risk of the sensitivity.

I sat and watched the continual downward spiral of his condition. The soy formula was being pumped into his stomach, and several times per day he would regurgitate it into his tracheotomy tubes and it would get into the ventilator tubes and sometimes go back to his lungs. This caused many complications and literally caused him to nearly choke to death. He was resuscitated twice. I kept telling the doctors, and they kept trying to reassure me that he needed this food. I respected their judgment, but I persisted because I believed the soy was causing problems. I knew it in my gut. I knew I could not let it go because I was the only one who could fight for this. I had to stand up for what I believed to be true. One of my husband's nurses was particularly compassionate, and she saw me growing weary. I was losing hope that he would recover.

One day I told that nurse how he had survived the accident, the surgeries, complications, and infections, and the soybeans were going to kill him. She walked out of the room and went directly over to her computer. Within a half hour, a new team of people I had not seen before came into the room. One was a dietician, and they immediately started to disconnect his feeding tube. She told me that they were going to figure out a new food since he had a soy allergy.

The nurse may have gotten in trouble if anyone else had noticed what she did. I believe the action she took that day saved his life. That evening, they began feeding him a new soy-free baby formula. He had a very good night and the next day began to improve. I walked out of the hospital feeling victorious in a very small but satisfying way.

Life threw another curveball. Just two weeks after my husband's forty-seven days in the hospital, our son and his friend were in a motorcycle accident. In case I hadn't learned enough about the value of traditional medicine, life was getting my attention.

While I learned that I needed to surrender to the judgment of the doctors and medical professionals, I also realized the value of trusting my gut and standing firmly to what I believed.

## Lesson Learned

I grew up with a hardcore attitude of conforming to the system and following your doctor's treatment protocol. I believed doctors were responsible for my health and well-being. I believed the holistic approach was unproven and risky. This was due to my ignorance.

Over the course of twenty years, I completely reversed my beliefs. The twists of fate with my own health led me to realize that medicine was harming me. I believe if I had continued on that path of managing my illnesses, I would have continued on that downward spiral. This led me to believe the "system" only managed disease and did not care about the long-term health of the patient. I found myself judging the whole system, its drug pushing and treating symptoms rather than finding causes and healing people. I completely shut myself off from the medical field.

While I walked into this hospital situation from a place of judgment, my husband's accident made me realize that nothing I could have done from a holistic standpoint could have saved his life. In his condition, there was nothing he could have done that would have kept him alive. Over the twenty-seven days in the ICU, I developed a deeper level of respect and appreciation for traditional medicine. I began to understand that most doctors have devoted their lives to helping their patients in the best way that they know how and with what they believe to be true based on their extensive training.

I was in the process of rebuilding my life as a single mom and needed extra income. I had been out of the laboratory for a number of years, and after the time I spent in the hospital, I was intrigued to learn more about medicine.

In addition to my speaking and coaching practice, I took a part-time job at a funeral home, enrolled in a medical terminology class, and became a certified Healthcare Technology Specialist for Practice Workflow and Redesign and a medical assistant. I now live in both worlds. I run my own practices in investigative health coaching for people and animals while also working as a part-time medical assistant. I feel I can best use my gifts and insights to serve humanity and help people learn how to heal when I understand both sides of the spectrum. It is my highest hope that I can help you heal all areas of your life by shedding light on the fact that we need both traditional medicine and holistic care to achieve a high level of well-being and to live lives in which we are enthused to wake up each day and experience all life has to offer.

## What Can We Learn about Health from Our Car?

We sometimes take better care of our car than we do of our bodies. We take it seriously when the check-engine light illuminates on our dashboard. We would not consider going on an extended road trip with the light on without having it first checked out and addressing the problem. On most occasions, we also regularly take our vehicle in for maintenance to ensure it runs smoothly. We don't just go to the serviceman and ask him to turn the check-engine light off without actually correcting the problem. It would be ridiculous to consider doing this without expecting a major malfunction to eventually occur. However, we often do this to our bodies. We feed ourselves poorly, and when a symptom shows up, we often neglect it, or we go to the doctor and have him remove a part or medicate it to stop the symptom. It takes care of the symptom but doesn't address the cause. Our symptoms are versions of our check-engine lights. They are a system that is in place to warn us that something is wrong. In reality, something we are doing or not doing is causing the system to malfunction.

Most of us would not feel comfortable putting substandard or contaminated oil or gasoline into our car in fear that it might damage the engine. Yet, as a society, many of us are eating substandard food. We eat fast food, junk food, and chemically processed food. The fact that this food has been approved as safe to eat and provides calories and energy doesn't mean it won't cause harm. This food is not contributing to our health, and it is damaging our bodies over the long term.

We have all heard the phrase, "An apple a day keeps the doctor away." This would ideally be an organic apple. I interpret this as meaning that if we consistently feed our bodies nutritious living food, we will not need to visit the doctor for a health crisis. Making healthy, informed choices is your best insurance of having a healthy body. This also goes for our minds. It is about preventive maintenance. We expect to do preventive maintenance on our cars. We change the oil, check the tire wear and pressure, fluid levels, the timing, and we periodically take it in for a tune-up to ensure everything is running well.

In my coaching practice, I focus on the "tune-up" aspect of our bodies. I look at what the body needs that traditional medicine may be missing, the lifestyle choices one is making, the sensitivities that may be causing disharmony in the body, and the environmental and emotional stressors that are keeping you from living a life of joy and purpose. Now, more than ever, we should work to be proactive about our health. We shouldn't wait until the system breaks down to try to fix it. It takes a lot of courage to take responsibility for our health. However, it is the only way to truly thrive.

In the first section of this book, "The Body and the Importance of Making Informed Choices," we will explore the body's ability to heal. I will share my expertise on important considerations you must take into account when choosing food and what you need to know about water quality, radiation, and the toxins to which you are exposed. I will then share with you some truths about scientific studies, the flaws of medicine, and how the desire for profits affects the health of our food supply and our bodies. We will also explore our impact on and responsibility to be stewards of the environment. We must learn some difficult truths about our toxic load in order to make informed choices and be empowered to fully support our bodies.

In the second section, "Mindset, Miracles, and the Spiritual Nature of Healing," we will explore how holistic practices can help us find and release the causes of disharmony in our bodies. I will share the fundamentals of healing that I have found through my experiences and in almost two decades working in the healing arts. Forgiving the system, the past, and, of course, ourselves will help us find the freedom to move on and experience life from a place of true well-being. We will focus on the missing components of healing, the power of belief, and the importance of self-care and implementing spiritual practices into our life.

In the final section, "The Bridge on the Path to Wellness," we will discuss the importance of integrating body health with spiritual and emotional well-being. Taking care of just the mind or the body without taking care of the other does not serve us in the long term. We are finding that true wellness only occurs if we nurture and support both our bodies *and* minds. Bridging science and spirituality, traditional medicine and holistic modalities, and being flexible is the best, easiest, most fulfilling way to heal and get the best return on investment. It is not about choosing one over the other. Bridging the gap between two worlds, thought processes, and philosophies will best serve humanity at this time. It is about balance and creating our best life.

# Chapter 2

# You Are the Healer

The essence of healing begins with you. You have more healing power than you might realize. It is important not to leave your healing entirely up to your medical team, God, or anyone else. In this chapter, I will discuss the value of listening to your symptoms, being open to different healing options, and taking responsibility for your healing.

## Let My Doctor Fix Me When I'm Broken

Illness is a process, and so is healing. You don't go to bed one night healthy and wake up the next morning with a disease. Over time, our choices affect our health. We have a tendency to seek disease-care instead of health-care. The model in which we exist treats symptoms instead of finding and correcting the root cause of illnesses, such as hidden toxins in our food, water, environment, or emotional stressors, sensitivities, and nutritional deficiencies. Fortunately, traditional medicine is extremely competent and is often capable of fixing you when you are broken. It remains the best option for acute problems.

Waiting for your system to break down is not the best option. You have the opportunity to protect and enhance your health. Remember the cliché "An ounce of prevention is worth a pound of cure." It is important to take responsibility for finding solutions and turning your life around after a malfunction, or you may relapse into a state of disease.

Would you put a gallon of milk or a bottle of soda into your gas tank and expect your car to operate properly? Your car's engine is not designed to operate on milk or soda. You wouldn't do this because you know it would cause the system to break down. Yet we often ingest food or beverages that our bodies are not designed to digest. Most of us know that we ingest things that are not good for us, yet we do it anyway. While it is important that we are not so rigid with ourselves that we can't enjoy life, we must also be conscientious of the impact our choices have on our bodies.

One evening as my family and I were at an auto racetrack, we witnessed a woman park her stroller in front of the bleachers. She proceeded to pour a can of cola into a bottle and hand it to her baby. We can agree there is no nutritional value in soda. There is no possible benefit to the baby unless it has become a habit and the baby is gratified because it has developed an addiction to the soda. If we studied that soda's ingredients, we would find that while the drink is approved for human consumption, it has ingredients that are toxic to the body, especially to that of a developing child. I would go so far as to say that some of the ingredients are neurotoxins and could be considered poisons.

My intention is not to judge or condemn this woman, but

to point out that each of us makes choices every day that impact our health. Her decision to give her baby soda will have consequences. If it were an isolated incident, the baby's body would most likely detoxify the soda. We would not expect to see any symptoms. What if she provided soda to this baby a few times per month? Weekly? Daily? The risk of developing a problem increases every time we repeat this behavior. Would you give your baby just a little bit of poison?

A number of things affect your health. These include nutrition, emotional and environmental stress, sensitivities, personal care products, deficiencies, the clothing you wear, and the amount of sleep you get. In this case, ignorance is not bliss. It is dangerous. There are consequences of eating food and using products that are not good for you.

In the coming chapters I will expose some problems in traditional medicine, our food supply, and our environment that are putting our health at risk. The things that I share are not obvious to the majority of the population because they are not recognized in the mainstream but may be causing your body distress right now. I will then lead you on a dedicated and focused journey to take your power back by looking within and asking the appropriate questions so you can take simple steps toward healing. I will also share practical ways to implement ancient healing principles that have been lost over time and share those missing components of healing, which as a society we are failing to incorporate into our lives.

## Symptoms

Behind every symptom you experience is a reason. They are not body malfunctions. They are there to caution you. They are an early-warning system of dis-ease or disharmony in your body. Sometimes the symptoms get louder or intensify to get our attention.

Don't ignore these symptoms. Covering them up or suppressing them will not fix the problem. This often makes the problem worse.

For example, consider pain medication. In the event of an injury, such as a sprain or fracture, I believe it could be used to give the body a break from the pain so you can relax and sleep peacefully. Your body has created the pain for a reason. There is an injury that requires rest so healing can occur. When you use the injured area a certain way, your level of pain will increase. This is your body's way of telling you that the movement is causing harm. If you take high doses of pain meds so that you don't feel the pain, you will likely go back to your normal activities and may cause further injury or inhibit healing.

Once, I took one of my teenage sons to the emergency room to evaluate a sports injury. After taking a look at him, the nurse offered him pain meds. He refused them. I honored my son's wisdom and his realization that he wanted to know how bad the pain was and to accurately describe the pain to the doctor who would eventually come in the room to examine the injury. The nurse appeared frustrated, told him he would not get a medal for enduring pain, and turned to me to see if I would overturn his decision. I stood by my son.

Trust your judgment. If you think you may have a broken bone, need stitches, or are experiencing chest pain or symptoms of a potentially serious acute condition, get to your nearest emergency room.

There are different ways to address symptoms. Traditional medicine often suppresses them. Alternative medicine works with the symptoms. Homeopathy is a perfect example of this. Let's say you have a fever. A fever is your body's natural way of heating up to kill off a pathogen. It is the way we were designed. Traditional medicine generally gives an over-the-counter drug to suppress the fever. It successfully lowers it into a normal temperature range. When the fever is suppressed, it is going against the body's natural process of heating up to kill off a pathogen. You may feel better because you do not have the symptoms associated with the fever. However, the pathogen is not eliminated. Sometimes the fever returns when the drug wears off after a few hours, and you have to take additional doses of the drug while your body fights the invader. Your body keeps trying to raise its temperature to eliminate the pathogen. You may even be given an antibiotic or antiviral drug because now your body's natural defense has been deactivated by suppressing the fever. This process might not necessarily be the best thing for you in the long run.

In homeopathy, an alternative therapy, a remedy is offered to increase the fever. This works with the body to assist in doing what the body was created to do. The fever generally spikes very rapidly for a short time and then returns to a normal temperature. This assists the body in killing off the bacteria or virus that has invaded you. The spike in temperature generally makes you feel worse, but it does not last long and successfully eliminates the pathogen and the need for drugs. You are back to feeling normal very quickly. In my experience the fever will spike for between ten and forty minutes after taking the homeopathic remedy, and you will be back to feeling well in just a few hours.

While these are two contrasting schools of thought on how to treat an illness or virus, they both have their place in our society. Homeopathy is a very interesting science and has been used for hundreds of years, well before pharmaceutical drugs entered the equation. It is mysterious and widely misunderstood because the remedies are dilutions of items that normally cause reactions. It is not necessary to understand how it works. It is a matter of understanding your options and weighing which option is best for you.

**Taking Responsibility**

I don't have the cleanest diet, but I make an effort to know the dangers of what I am eating, am aware of my sensitivities, and make each choice a conscious, well-informed one. After paying close attention for many years, I know how my bad choices affect me. If I eat GMO food ingredients, I will have heartburn. If I eat wheat, I will gain weight. If I am in contact with bleach or fabrics that have been bleached, I will get hives. If I eat food dyes, I will likely break out in a rash within a few days. I know my body. If I eat chemical preservatives, artificial sweeteners, or cinnamon, I will get a headache. I also get a headache and become irritable when I am exposed to perfumed products such as laundry detergents, cologne, air fresheners, or scented candles. If I experience any of those symptoms, I can trace it back and figure out what I did that caused it. It is not that my body just randomly gave me a headache or broke out in hives. There is a connection between what we ingest and how we feel.

So many of us believe we will just do whatever we want and rely on our doctors to reverse the damage. Others do their best to optimize their health and avoid the need for medical intervention and dependence on long-term drug use to fight the symptoms. While drugs have become very advanced at targeting specific areas and processes in the body, there is still collateral damage caused from taking a drug.

Your health is your responsibility. Illness is a result of conscious choices or ignorance. You either knowingly or unknowingly contribute to the problem. You are not a victim. You do not catch disease by some misfortune. You create the conditions for them to occur with poor diet, water, or air quality, infections or dental toxins, or by dwelling on stress, drama, fears, or negativity.

There is always a lesson in or insight into every illness and symptom. There are several stories in this book that will illustrate this point. But the greatest takeaway for you should be to maintain a willingness to listen and learn from them. If you were to really listen, what is your body telling you?

**Everything Is Energy**

Most of my books start with the fact that everything is energy. When you balance your energy and raise your vibration, you change your life. Balancing your energy has the most profound impact on your well-being. East Asian cultures have understood this for thousands of years. Western medicine is slow to embrace the possibilities that exist when we look at the energetic body. In Western medicine, anatomy and physiology are taught by studying cadavers, which have no life-force energy. No element of life-force energy can be dissected from a cadaver or seen under a microscope, so it is often dismissed.

The intention of this book is not to prove scientific facts or debate religion. It is not meant to sway you to any one perspective. It is intended to help you open your mind and your heart and explore the possibilities of the unlimited potential you have within. We are more than our physical bodies. Everyone has the capacity to heal and the ability to summon and welcome miracles.

I admire your courage and willingness to learn, to take responsibility, to read this book, to ask questions, and to take a proactive role to heal your life.

When we get our minds and our bodies into a state of homeostasis and energetic balance, all healing is possible. When this is widely understood, we will see a healing revolution.

### The Body's Innate Wisdom

As demonstrated with the fundamental example of having a fever, the body has an incredible ability to bounce back from insult and heal itself when given a chance. All forms of life are miraculous. There is an innate wisdom that is beyond the comprehension of the human mind. Science may never understand or be able to define or replicate the wisdom of nature or God.

While we would like to consider ourselves to know it all, we are very limited in our understanding and you will see evidence of this as the years unfold. Healing is continuously happening throughout the body. Billions of cells in your body are replaced every day. Your body is constantly working to heal itself.

Our bodies adapt and can withstand constant insult

from pesticides, pathogens, and other negative environmental, emotional, and dietary factors. Our habits, actions, and choices disrupt the healing process, create the disease, or the conditions which support it. Some have a strong constitution and can cope for a period of time. No one knows what that period will be before the system begins to break down.

We create our own limitations in life and in healing. If you view diseases differently, you have different choices to heal them.

## Only God Can Heal

During a keynote presentation, I indicated that the body has an incredible ability to heal itself. I later found out that a woman in the audience walked out after I made that statement. One of the sponsors approached her and asked if everything was alright. She stated that she was leaving because no one has the ability to heal themselves and that only God can heal anyone. The woman left the event, and I was never able to meet her or address her concern.

My intention when I do a presentation is to inform, inspire, and empower my audience. I do not want to leave them in a place of judgment and discontent. When this sort of thing happens in my event, I want to explore it. It could simply be this person's own projections and fears. In some cases a person is simply not willing to hear the perspective of another. I understand that not everyone will be open to hear what I have to say. Some will outright disagree with me. That is fine. We have our own beliefs. If I am teaching something that is wrong or causes frustration, I want to take responsibility for that and make amends where appropriate. We are all on a journey to discover what is true for us. There is a reason that it came up in my event. I recognized there is something in it for me to learn. If I were to dismiss her comment, I would be doing my audiences from that point forward a disservice. I would also fail to explore an issue that was intended for me. I have learned to trust that life is giving me exactly what I need in every moment. The fact that I was made aware of this tells me that there is something I need to learn from it or teach about it. Be open to seeing the messages that are intended for you.

I want to address her concern and share my thoughts. Her comment brought up many personal questions. I spent my flight home contemplating the relationship between God and healing. When a child falls and skins her knee, doesn't her mother's hug begin her healing? Isn't God within all of us? Did He not create us in his own likeness? If He does not bestow the powers to heal upon humans, then why do we go to doctors expecting to be healed? Would it be wrong for someone to go to a doctor seeking medical treatment if they believe strongly that only God can heal?

Did God intend that only certain saints, prophets, or angels could perform miracles? Are we not all created equally? There is a part of each of us that is divine. Every cell in our bodies is divine. At some level, we are all a bit afraid of our magnificence. We are a society that is using only 5 percent of our brains. We understand just a small fraction of how things work.

Religion is often viewed as the destination. I believe this is a misconception. The purpose of life is the evolution of the soul. It is all about the journey and who we become in the process.

I have come to believe that religion is simply a path to God. It consists of rituals, a community, and the celebration of faith. We get caught up in focusing on the path.

God is an issue of faith, not religion. Science cannot prove God. We all experience God a little differently. For some of us, God is the only truth and the only way. Many live their lives in devotion to God, many have given their lives in religious wars, and for many, faith in God has gotten them through their toughest challenges. To that end, healing is an issue of faith. There is a mystical aspect of healing that science does not understand.

We hold strong beliefs for years that often are later proved to be wrong. Evolving in our beliefs occurs in a natural order as our understanding and life experiences expand. It is human nature to be skeptical. Early in our lives, we have all been deceived. Becoming skeptical is a protective measure we take at a subconscious level to prevent ourselves from being taken advantage of or of being made a fool.

From the deepest place in my soul, I believe the power of healing is within each of us. I believe you are more capable of healing than you realize. I believe that thinking we cannot heal goes against what God intends for us to be. Ask God or the universe for what you need. Embrace the fact that God never fails. Look inward instead of outside for all of the answers. Work to have an attitude of gratitude. Give thanks for your healing and for the harmony and balance in your body.

**Lessons from Cancer**

I've lost a number of family members and a close friend to cancer. My closest experience was with my father. He had cancer twice. When he was diagnosed with colon cancer the first time at age fifty, he had surgery to remove it. He wasn't open to chemotherapy or radiation. I lived out of state, so I wasn't close to the day-to-day occurrences. It was difficult living far away, and I did not feel at all influential in any of the choices that were made. I was merely a bystander from afar.

My father survived and was cancer free for ten years before it returned. It was the same cancer from a decade before. This time it metastasized. It was first in his lungs and later in his brain and bones. He was still resistant to doing chemo or radiation. I truly believed he would be giving up if he didn't undertake the recommended treatment. I urged him to do it because at that time I believed it was the best solution and the only way that he would survive the disease. This second time he had cancer, I lived only a few miles away, so I was there for him and my family and physically present several times a week. He chose to go through with the chemo and radiation. For the most part, it was a physical and emotional rollercoaster of hope and despair.

If my father had chosen chemotherapy or radiation when he had cancer the first time, who knows if he would have survived. No expert on this planet could say for certain. Perhaps the treatment would have led to his death that time. I may be judged for making that statement, but in my heart, it is the truth. There is also the question of if he had undergone chemo for cancer the first time, would it have prevented the cancer from returning? Is it possible that he may have survived the second incidence with cancer if he had not done the chemo and radiation treatment?

No one will ever know the answer to those questions. One thing is for certain: Having those ten extra years allowed him many additional experiences in life, like meeting his grandchildren. The joy he experienced from spending time with his grandsons has left a profound imprint on our hearts.

I've learned a lot from that experience. Looking back, I regret that I urged my dad to do chemotherapy. I wanted him to follow allopathic medicine because that was all I knew. I was conditioned to believe that chemotherapy was the only answer. I believed that he would die if he did not do it. It was a fear-based decision, and I have changed my viewpoint over the years. If I knew then what I know now, I would not have urged him to undergo chemotherapy or radiation.

I now choose to honor a person's choice of treatment. If a person decides not to do chemo, it doesn't mean they've given up and that death is imminent. Our bodies were created with an innate wisdom to heal. It is possible that many people have a better chance of survival without chemo or intervention as long as they address the cause of their disease.

Each one of us is in a unique place and has his or her own set of beliefs. We have different levels of trust in our gut feelings. We've had different experiences. We've had different exposures. We have different body chemistries and constitutions. We're not going to respond the same way to any given treatment.

What's right for one person is not necessarily right for another. I don't think there's one other medical case that is exactly the same as yours. Your treatment plan and ability to recover has nothing to do with anyone else's experience. Ultimately, it's up to each person to decide what feels right for him or her when faced with treatment choices. We each have our own journey to live. Some of my clients with cancer have decided not to tell their families about it. They don't want the pressure, the drama, or the burden of additional fears or negativity, and I completely understand and honor that choice now.

I have recently changed my viewpoint on obtaining a diagnosis. Not everyone needs one. We will explore the impact of a diagnosis later in this book. Sometimes, symptoms and the fear of not knowing what is happening with your body can cause tremendous stress. In this event, a diagnosis is warranted. Each case is different. At times you need to rule something out, or you may need to get a baseline so you can track your progress. Do what feels right to you. If you have physical symptoms that are not resolving or that you feel are serious, or you feel emotionally out of control, by all means seek medical help. In many cases, it is the best option. We've gotten lost in fear and turned our power over to others. Some have worked hard to condition us or convince us to believe what they want us to believe.

While there are great drugs to mask your pain and suppress your symptoms, there is still a lot of unnecessary suffering and short- and long-term consequences of treatment. If you are currently undergoing treatment for any condition, ask yourself if it is enhancing your life. If the treatment is necessary to boost your quality of life, think of it as a temporary plan. Always seek a better way.

I have been doing sensitivity screenings since 1999. It is amazing to witness the dramatic shift in people's symptoms simply by avoiding food they are sensitive to. Many people heal simply by avoiding things that are not good for them. The body heals when the burden is eliminated.

While I have used herbal and homeopathic remedies, it is important to note that herbal preparations and some alternative therapies may interfere with the effectiveness or have a negative reaction with your medications. Herbal remedies can also affect blood pressure, thin the blood or affect clotting, and have dangerous consequences during pregnancy. You should seek medical advice and discuss your protocols with your doctor. Do not blindly accept everything you read on the Internet. Assemble a team of doctors and practitioners that respect your beliefs and listen to you.

**And in the End . . .**

We really don't know the exact effect of any specific treatment. There are so many variables. It is assumed that if someone improves from a treatment, then the treatment is credited for the healing. We do not know if the person's beliefs, diet, time, or other factors played a role in their physical improvement. When something "worked," we don't know if a different treatment option would have worked better or would be more lasting. We will never know. We make the choice of how to handle an illness, disease or symptom, and proceed.

If someone undergoes a treatment and does not get better, it does not mean that treatment will not work for someone else. Sometimes, people think it was too late or they may have been one of the unfortunate members of that percentage of people that a specific treatment does not work for. Your body may not be healing because of something you are exposing it to. This chapter is designed to help you better understand that you play a tremendous role in your health and if necessary, in your healing. Do your due diligence and investigate all forms of medicine and lifestyle changes to ensure you are taking the correct path for you. Don't limit yourself to seeing a doctor and then blindly following "the plan." Take your health seriously. The food you introduce into your body and the environment you surround yourself with can keep you healthy or unhealthy for years to come. In the end, there is no better healer than you.

The following chapters will help you identify things that may be harming you that you may not be aware of. They will also help you make more informed choices. It will serve you to pay attention to those things that stand out. They are getting your attention for a reason. Commit to making a few small changes to get or stay healthy.

# Chapter 3

# Flaws in the Medical System

To stay healthy, you must understand how and where medicine fails us. This chapter will focus on exposing some of the problems in medicine. This includes the push to medicate symptoms instead of finding solutions, how money drives the pharmaceutical industry, and how fear keeps it all working. I will discuss my experiences as a research scientist and how study results are skewed in favor of those with a financial interest in the outcome. I will also explain the risks of being in the hospital and of medical treatment, the dangers of screening tests, the cholesterol myth, and the high cost of healthcare that is keeping some people from seeking treatment.

## Managing Disease

Traditional medicine has brilliant diagnostic abilities, intervention, emergency, and trauma care. They save many lives in those areas every day. One role of traditional medicine is to manage chronic disease. Disease care is not healthcare. It may keep you alive, but it does not keep you healthy. Having worked in research, health, and medicine for the majority of my career, camped out in hospitals and watching treatment protocols with the keen eye of a scientist, who has no special interest other than to understand and make sense of it all, I would say that you are best off using your time, effort, and money to stay healthy rather than to fight off disease. My work is about improving the quality of life by optimizing health and well-being through education and empowerment. My intention is to arm you with enough information to empower you to take control of those areas of your life.

The system is not designed to cure chronic conditions but to manage them. The model supports a diagnosis that will lead to either a procedure or extended medication that will need to be monitored for life.

When you only treat a symptom, over the long term you will generally create more problems than you solve. Many drugs have toxic ingredients and are harmful to the body. That is why they work. Do not depend on pharmaceutical drugs over the long term if you can correct the problem by finding the root cause and changing your diet, lifestyle, emotional state, and mindset.

Traditional medicine usually treats a problem or symptom as exclusive. There is sometimes a pill for each symptom. They don't look at the body as a whole. I am not saying there is not a time and place for drugs. I believe there are many times when drugs are warranted over the short term. The problem is that we have become a society taking a large number of drugs in combinations that have never been studied. Patients often see multiple doctors who prescribe different drugs. Some doctors don't want to take a patient off a drug. Once a patient starts to take a particular medication, unless they are having a noticeable adverse reaction, or ask their doctor to stop it, they generally remain on it. I see patients come in with a shopping bag full of drugs, with a multitude of symptoms, sometimes not knowing why they are taking certain drugs, taking drugs to manage the side effects of other drugs, and wondering why they feel terrible all the time. As a society, we must realize that health does not come from a pill.

Sadly, factors drive the way medicine is practiced that are not always in our best interest. It is a broken mindset. There are motives that extend beyond the greater good of mankind. It is a great business model if your main objective is to make money.

Doctors have the highest level of integrity and want the best outcome for their patients. Doctors have your best interest at heart. They are doing the best they can with what they believe, with what they have been taught, and while staying within the scope of their license.

Medical students are taught that a drug protocol can fix almost any problem. From a pharmaceutical perspective, we are biochemical beings that can be chemically altered by these drugs in order to regulate our symptoms. Pharmaceutical companies sponsor most medical schools. Medical schools teach how to prescribe patented drugs. The curriculum is developed by paid drug company instructors. Physicians have been trained by special interests to believe and behave a specific way.

The bottom line for drug companies is shareholder return. They make money if a patient starts a new drug or remains on a drug. They lose money if the patient is cured and no longer needs the drug. As publicly held corporations, they have to answer to their shareholders and not to God. The problem becomes that drug companies run the medical schools, do their own research, subsidize the training, censor the content of medical journals, and sponsor the medical symposiums. A drug's success is not generally measured by its effectiveness to cure illness, but by how much money it generates for its manufacturer.

After working on high-level research projects and understanding the role of statistical analysis, I have learned to be very skeptical of research studies that are conducted by any group, person, corporation, or organization that has any financial ties to the outcome. Studies can be easily manipulated to prove any outcome that you desire, and they are often rigged to avoid finding problems. Tragically, many proven facts are based on bias and can just as easily be disproven. The same data can be used to prove or disprove a theory simply based on which statistical tool is used to analyze the data.

It is hard for these tests to appear objective when there is a vested interest in the outcome. To dive deeper, it is important to consider a number of questions. Who did the study? Who funded the study? Who benefits from the sale of the drug or procedure being tested? Who has the vested interest in the outcome? Studies must be designed ethically and responsibly with true control groups by someone with no financial interests.

A research study is summarized in an abstract that appears at the beginning of the study. The abstract, which gives a brief overview of the study with conclusions, is often the only part of a research report that anyone reads. It is often not a true representation of what the study concluded.

Medicine puts their faith in randomized, double-blind, placebo-controlled, peer-reviewed studies that are sponsored, conducted, or funded by those with a vested interest in the outcome. They discredit all other studies. The result is that many doctors don't realize how biased their training and education is to focus on treatments that yield great profits to those who trained them. I know many well-intentioned medical professionals and drug company representatives. I fully believe they are doing their jobs to the best of their ability in accordance with the training they have received. They believe they are contributing to the well-being of society by offering these drugs. This is their truth.

## The Consequences of the Medical Model

Medicine today largely separates the mind, energetic body or spirit, and mouth from the physical body. It has forgotten that separating them limits our capacity to heal. Traditional medicine treats the physical body and often overlooks the other components. When we look at the study of anatomy, most of what is known about the body comes from the study of cadavers. It does not take into account anything more. Energy meridians cannot be seen anatomically and will not be found upon dissection. It does not acknowledge an energetic body, the effect of intention and belief, or a vital life-force energy that might have a larger influence on the body than its physiological processes. East Asian medicine and ancient cultures have understood this for thousands of years.

While medicine studies the body through the dissection of cadavers, from my experience of looking at the body from a holistic perspective, I feel that traditional, allopathic medicine is the best way to obtain a diagnosis. Once you get the diagnosis, it is up to you to accept it and become defeated by it, or to find a better way to deal with it, handle it, live with it, or heal it. Traditional medicine is not always the best path for finding the cause of the problem. Sometimes it offers incredibly quick ways to treat and stop the symptoms, which do not always heal the body. They provide relief to the patient, which is often desperately needed. So often I find that people end up managing their diseases for many years without ever figuring out why they have them in the first place.

Medical interventions can save, prolong, and improve

the quality of your life. I urge you to use them when you need to. The standardization of healthcare is not working as well as we think. We are individuals and will respond differently to our food, environment, and stress. We will respond in a unique manner to each treatment. While the cookie-cutter approach may serve society as a whole, it does not look at you as an individual.

The United States has a higher cost of healthcare than almost all other countries while still ranking low for efficiency, quality of care, and health. According to The Commonwealth Fund and World Health Organization, Americans have shorter life expectancies and more chronic conditions compared to most other nations. Life expectancy numbers are skewed because of the sharp decline in infant mortality due to advancements in neonatal care, increases in survival rates due to efficient trauma care, and medical interventions. We are not living longer, and our quality of life in our senior years is decreasing.

Something is profoundly wrong with science when short-term political gains, personal bonuses, and profits become more important than truth and the advancement of science, health, and healing. Often when people acknowledge this, they are discredited, shamed, and lose their jobs.

Medical professionals are under tremendous pressure to conform to the system. In some cases, if they suggest "alternative" treatments they jeopardize the very license that they worked so hard to get. This creates tremendous fear and ensures they will stay with the protocol they are taught.

I had an interesting experience where I conducted tapping sessions with a man who had serious emotional issues after a long history of abuse. For those who have never heard of tapping, it is a form of emotional acupressure that effectively releases negative emotions. After each session, I gave a summary to his doctor. The doctor was impressed with the level of understanding I had with this man and the direction our sessions took. The doctor suggested I go back to school and get licensed in some form of therapy so I could bill insurance. I believe he was quite surprised when I told him I would not get licensed because I knew that once I adopted a title, there would be rules that govern that title and I would be required to work by those rules and follow protocols. That is not always in the best interest of the patient because it takes away the creativity of the practitioner and does not allow for much thinking outside the box.

Government and industries mandate our healthcare. Government should not be allowed to mandate our healthcare choices. It should not be able to detain us or prohibit our children from attending school if they don't comply unless they are an actual threat to the well-being of others. The word *actual* is key here.

Most insurance companies will not cover anything outside protocol but will cover routine procedures. I don't do mammograms. I don't take synthetic drugs. I don't get flu shots. I won't be having any more babies. So I feel I pay for this insurance and don't use the routine benefits that they offer as standard care. They pay to find things wrong with you, to manage your problems, but not to keep you healthy or fix chronic problems.

With changes that have occurred in the health insurance industry, insurance premiums are going up and the coverage is going down. Many of us are forced to choose treatments, tests, and medications based on financial ability. I live this personally. I have a high annual deductible because I don't use medical treatments often. At the time of this writing, my premium is more than $7,000 per year for two, and we each have a deductible of $7,200 plus a $1,000 copay each time we visit an emergency room. I recently had a health issue, and I contemplated going in for evaluation. I knew which tests would need to be run to reach a diagnosis and that the cost of them would eat up my deductible. I could not justify paying $8,200 out of pocket before my insurance kicked in, so I opted not to seek treatment.

In reality, no one wants to spend $8,200 to find out indigestion, stress, or having eaten too much salt caused their spike in blood pressure or chest palpitations. That financial burden does not fit into the budget of a single parent, a young person just getting established in life, or a senior citizen on a fixed income. Many people tell me they are in this same predicament. It is causing a lot of us to make our own preliminary health assessments and keeping some of us from seeking immediate medical care for a symptom that could potentially be serious.

Millions of people are struggling with prescription drug addictions. Experts agree that about 2 percent of the American population is addicted to prescription painkillers. According to *Scientific American*, one in six people are taking a psychiatric drug. According to the Foundation for a Drug-Free World, more than fifteen million Americans abuse prescription drugs. Prescription drugs kill more people than street drugs.

Pharmaceutical companies are advertising directly to the patient now. Turn on any primetime-television show and you are likely to see a number of advertisements for the latest, greatest drugs. Patients can go into their doctor's office asking for the drug, already convinced that it might help them. If the doctor doesn't see any problem or contraindications, he or she may prescribe the drug. If the patient hadn't seen the commercial, he may never have been prescribed this drug in the first place.

Teachers are essentially diagnosing students with attention disorders. I have seen this happen many times. Teachers advise parents to take their child to their doctor because of an attention issue. In many cases the doctor will then prescribe medication for the child because the parent comes in convinced that the child has an attention problem. I think these drugs are some of the most overprescribed and dangerous. They are numbing out a generation of children. Children don't feel anxious, but they also don't feel joy. I believe they are altering brain chemistry and causing many children to act out irrationally. The side effects are causing mental and emotional instability.

In a drug-based model, some doctors receive a commission based on the treatment they provide. In any business there is a benefit to upselling additional products or services. Even holistic practitioners make money off the services or supplements they provide. Many oncologists receive commission on chemotherapy drugs. The more drugs they sell, the more patients they convince to go on chemotherapy, the more money they make.

Consider the fact that many chemotherapy drugs are carcinogens. They cause cancer. Mammograms emit ionizing radiation, which is one of the main causes of breast cancer. The very tests that are used to detect cancer cause cancer. The very treatment to kill cancer causes cancer. When cancer "comes back" a few years after a "successful" treatment, I can't help but wonder if this "new" cancer is from the treatment itself.

I met a chiropractor whose thirteen-year-old daughter had been diagnosed with cancer. He did not believe that chemotherapy would be her best treatment option, and they opted to take a more holistic route. He was threatened with his daughter being taken away by Child Protective Services and was told he would face charges of negligence and endangerment if he did not follow the prescribed treatment plan. They fought it the best that they could but were forced to put their daughter on chemotherapy. This medical standard of care does not give the patient any choice.

At the time of this writing, my mother is eighty-one and in great health. She was recently evaluated by a new doctor. She had no acute or new problems; she just needed to establish care with a new provider. The doctor told her she needed to stop most of her supplements and start a drug protocol. Taking supplements does not fit into any drug company protocol. My heart sank when I learned of this. Luckily, my mom preferred her way because it has been working for her. She refused the proposed plan.

My sister once saw a sign hanging in a doctor's office that said, "Don't confuse your Google search with my medical degree." I have seen doctors get defensive, humiliate patients, and discredit them for questioning the protocol. This is not the doctor you want. Find a doctor who truly respects your ability to think outside the box and does not belittle you because you think you know your body better than he or she does. Find a doctor who listens to you and who you feel cares deeply about your well-being even if that means you will no longer need to be "managed."

Keep in mind that doctors must protect themselves from litigation. If you refuse standard practices, they will need to document that and may even need to say you are noncompliant. Some doctors may refuse to see you if you do not comply with their directives. They may refuse to treat your children if you do not want to authorize a specific treatment for them. They may be doing you a favor. Find a doctor who honors you. There are many brilliant doctors who will listen to you and do the best they can to honor your beliefs and concerns.

## Stress

According to the American Psychological Association, 75 percent of doctor's visits are for complaints related to stress. Many scientific studies have proven that chronic stress is an underlying cause of illness and disease. Physiologically, stress can weaken the immune system, interfere with sleep cycles, raise inflammatory markers, affect blood flow, slow the digestive system, raise blood pressure, and cause emotional disorders, endocrine disruption, sexual dysfunction, diabetes, ulcers, heart disease, and cancer. Our bodies were created to adapt during periods of short-term stress. We were not designed to be under the constant stress created by our lifestyles.

Traditional medicine doesn't really have effective methods of helping people with stress. Talk therapy is helpful and has given many people the support they need, but even that must often continue for years or even decades since it takes time for people to find peace with the issues they face. Sadly, the most common treatments are antianxiety or antidepressant medications. Traditional medicine has a tendency to treat the mind mainly with drugs.

There are many effective techniques for managing stress. Some of my favorites are GetSet™ Tapping, mindful breathing, and meditation. These offer simple ways to quiet the mind, eliminate mental chatter, and bring inner peace while allowing one to accept themselves and their circumstances in the current moment. We will explore some of these in Section II.

### Fear and Stress Feed the System

Fear increases stress and potentially disease. It drives us to take determined action to keep us feeling safe. It also perpetuates profits for those who benefit from our fears. I met a woman on a flight who told me about her daughter and the adoption process she underwent. I asked her why she chose that particular route of adoption. She said that she was unable to have children because she had needed a hysterectomy. What she said next stunned me: She needed to have the hysterectomy, she said, because she was "going" to get cancer. She said that she had a routine pap test, which revealed precancerous cells. She was told if she didn't do something about it, she would have cancer within two years. I mustered every bit of strength I had to hold back from blurting, "Are you flippin' kidding me?" I thought, *How can someone project that? Is there a business motive behind this to make money off the surgery? Surely there is a less invasive way to monitor and heal this.*

Luckily this woman had the resources to adopt a child. Many women have shared with me that they did not have children because their medical team had warned them against it due to supposed risk factors. This has left many women without realizing one of their biggest dreams.

It breaks my heart. I myself was told that I might not be able to have children. Highly trained professionals shared with me that even if I did, I would have a very hard time getting pregnant. I was devastated because I believed what the doctor told me. This was just a few weeks before my wedding, and I had to have the difficult conversation with my husband-to-be. I was deeply saddened by this "fact." A month later, I was pregnant. I gave birth to three amazing baby boys over the next four years.

During one of my pregnancies, I was working as a quality assurance chemist and was about to lead a safety meeting for about one hundred employees when my phone rang. It was my obstetrician telling me that she needed to discuss the results of one of my screening tests—an alpha fetoprotein test that detects congenital abnormalities. My results indicated that my baby had a high probability of having Down syndrome. The next hour was a blur. I was devastated, and I didn't even remember what I said in the meeting.

I was sent for a consultation with a genetic counselor, which ended up being a coaching session about the feasibility of having a "medically necessary" abortion. I knew

I would not abort the baby so I didn't understand why we were having this meeting. I struggled with so many things in my mind. Was I capable of being the mother I needed to be for this child? This stress was not healthy for me or my baby. In the end I gave birth to a perfectly healthy boy.

I have since changed my views completely on screening tests. People may judge me for not doing screenings because they are led to believe that screening will save your life. They believe I am putting myself at risk.

When I was diagnosed with liver tumors, I explored alternatives. I found that the body has an incredible ability to heal itself if it's given what it needs. I often wonder how many of us have had cancer or other diseases and our bodies have healed without our ever being aware of its presence. It leads me to question the impact of early-detection screenings. It makes me wonder if we keep looking for something hard enough will we eventually find it? Will we cause problems by testing for them or by fearing that we have them? Is that what we truly want? Are screening tests truly advancing medicine? For whose benefit? Are they leading to more business for the industry that tells us how important it is to do the screening? I don't say that lightly. It is a deep concept to contemplate, and the answer will be different for everyone depending on where you are in your journey.

Good insurance that covers and encourages frequent early-detection screening tests is probably not the best thing for your health. Early-detection screenings are doing harm in terms of fear, stress, and physical consequences. Those need to be considered against the benefits. Regular screenings may be important for you. Finding and treating a problem in its early stages may be right for you. Know that you have options, and make the choice that is best for you.

We are conditioned to perceive things, formulate our beliefs, and act based on our programming. Water runs downhill and follows the path of least resistance. We tend to follow the path of least resistance with our choices. We do what is easiest and make choices based on what we know from our previous experiences. We follow the advice of others whom we respect and trust. We often take their advice blindly.

In my fifty some years on the planet, one thing I have found is that universal truth is very important to me. I cannot tolerate propaganda. For that reason, I do not watch the news. I do not waste my energy on things that suck the life out of me. Life is too precious. Do not get caught up in the hype. There is often an agenda, and fear is used to cause people to do irrational things and not even realize it. We have a tendency to believe that everything that is suggested to us is in our best interest. Use caution and trust your gut.

## Cholesterol Myth

My brother was seeking medical help for heartburn. They ran a battery of tests to monitor his stomach acid and blood chemistry. We sat one evening over a family dinner discussing his results. Our family has a history of elevated cholesterol, and we had been told that hypercholesterolemia, or high cholesterol, puts you at risk of heart disease. My brother was excited and relieved that his total serum cholesterol was one hundred sixty-three milligrams per deciliter, well within the low-risk level. He was perplexed because they could not find anything wrong. He was a strong, fit forty-one-year-old man who loved the outdoors and physical activity.

That was the last conversation I had with my brother. It was the last time my family and I saw my brother alive. Forty hours later, we received the dreadful call that he was dead. We were shocked, and we wanted answers. We had an autopsy performed. The cause of death was ruled an acute myocardial infarction, or heart attack due to almost complete blockage of the coronary arteries. How could this be? If cholesterol is an indication of blockage, why was his in the "perfect" range one week earlier?

Just recently, a friend who has his cholesterol monitored a couple of times per year with "perfect" numbers and never a value "out of range," had three successive surgeries to open complete blockages in multiple arteries. If his cholesterol level was so low, how could he have such substantial plaque on his artery walls?

In some countries, cholesterol is not considered a risk factor for cardiovascular events. I have studied different perspectives on the issue. Did God make a mistake and give us "bad" cholesterol? Are our bodies that were created with such precision malfunctioning? Could it be that the "bad" cholesterol is scavenging the blood and doing its job exactly as it intended to do? If the level of "bad" cholesterol is high, isn't that possibly an indication that it is doing what it is supposed to do and not an indication of risk, but rather that there is something else going on in the body causing this cholesterol to go into action?

As witnessed with my brother, we are led to put so much faith in these numbers. They really mean nothing. These numbers can put us in a state of fear or give us a false sense of security. They can drive us to take drugs such as statins, which can cause collateral damage in the body.

Statins are a class of widely prescribed drugs that interfere with cholesterol metabolism. Statins deplete coenzyme Q10 (CoQ10) from the body. If you are taking a statin drug to lower your cholesterol, ask your doctor about supplementing CoQ10. The rule of thumb is one milligram of CoQ10 per pound of body weight.

At one point my doctor's nurse called to tell me that my cholesterol tested high and the doctor wanted to prescribe a cholesterol-lowering drug. I refused the drug, but the doctor was never informed. I decided to work on lowering my cholesterol with an herbal tincture of guggul lipid. I went for another cholesterol test and a follow-up with my doctor. He said he was very impressed with how well the drug had lowered my cholesterol and had never seen such a drastic change in a short period. I told him that I did not take the drug and had taken an herb instead. He quickly said there must have been an error in the lab because it was impossible for the cholesterol to go down that quickly without a drug. I thought it was interesting that had I taken the drug, my reduced cholesterol level would have been credited to the drug; but now that I had revealed I had used an herb, my results were being discredited.

I no longer believe cholesterol is an indicator of heart attack risk. I could not find any studies that show that lowering your cholesterol reduces your chances of dying from a coronary event. The truth is our cells need cholesterol. It performs many vital functions in our bodies. Damaged cells absorb cholesterol. Cholesterol is essential for brain function, the nervous system, synthesis or neurotransmitters, and synthesis of vitamin D. Our liver was designed to make cholesterol. Cholesterol is not the problem. Research suggests low levels of cholesterol increase cancer risk. This is one of my biggest frustrations with medicine. The medical field is doing the best it can with the information that has been disseminated to it. It's human nature to believe what we are taught. But the truth is that simple discovery and information can lead you to new and much better paths to live a healthy lifestyle.

## Hospital Food

I accompanied a friend as an advocate for a spinal surgery. She was offered snacks upon coming out of the anesthesia. These snacks consisted of sandwich cookies, soft chocolate chip cookies, cheese-flavored crackers, soda, fruit juice, coffee, ice cream, and gelatin desserts. I took pictures of this "food" because I didn't think anyone would believe this story. There was nothing of any nutritional value offered at a time when the body is coming off the trauma of the drugs and surgery and needs to heal.

On a different occasion, I was in the hospital with a friend who was put on a cardiac diet after surgery. I was horrified by the food options that were part of this special diet. Meals frequently consisted of luncheon meat and cheese sandwiches, baked potato chips, sugary fruit juices, and canned soda. One meal consisted of a crispy catfish sandwich, pound cake with GMO margarine, decaffeinated coffee, and a packaged fruit cup. Another meal was a low-fat milk product and packaged cereal with white toast and GMO margarine. My body would have had a negative response if I had eaten one meal off that hospital tray. Just because something has been approved by the FDA or a governmental regulatory agency, recommended by a dietician, or sold as food, does not mean that it contributes to your health or well-being. The very place you expect to be nurtured back to health feeds you toxins.

Now when I visit a friend in the hospital, I will often bring food such as organic fruit or healthy choices instead of flowers. I make sure the hospital has not given them any dietary restrictions. I know the hospital food service will not provide the level of nutrition anyone needs to overcome the stress of being hospitalized, the trauma of the intervention, or the impact of the drugs.

## Hospital Errors

While hospitals are constantly striving to improve their error rates, errors do happen. You do not want to be one of the statistics.

According to the Centers for Disease Control and Prevention and Johns Hopkins Medicine, approximately 250,000 people die each year as a result of medical mistakes. This makes medical mistakes the third leading cause of death in the United States. A growing epidemic of burnout is sweeping the medical field. Medical professionals are under tremendous stress to follow guidelines, meet regulatory demands, and perform clerical tasks in addition to performing their duties of providing medical care. Changes in medicine are forcing many seasoned doctors to retire early, leaving the ones who stay on with the extra pressure of meeting the needs of more patients and picking up where the new medical students simply don't have the experience to treat complex cases.

Additionally, over one hundred thousand people in the United States die each year from adverse reactions to properly prescribed, properly dispensed, properly taken prescription drugs. This does not include mortality from people who were inadvertently put on the wrong drug, given the wrong drug by the pharmacy, or took it improperly. If you are one of the people who suffer the consequences of an adverse reaction to a drug or treatment, the problem is very real.

I have come to believe that anyone who has been sedated or is on narcotic pain medication needs an advocate by their side. I would never allow my loved one to be in the hospital without an advocate, even when it means camping out on a chair for days or weeks on end. I would rather be there to prevent something that is easily preventable and work on catching up on sleep when they are discharged.

Once when my father was in the hospital, his medications were accidentally given to his roommate. This caused the gentleman serious distress that could have threatened his life. On another occasion, I was in the hospital with my mom immediately after surgery and they brought her pain medication. She was still coming out of the anesthesia and was not yet coherent. A few minutes later, another nurse came in with a cup of medications. When I questioned the nurse about the medicine, I told her they had already given my mom those pills a few minutes prior.

We are all human and errors do happen. Patients are not always in the frame of mind to notice these problems, and medical staff doesn't always catch the errors. The medical staff may not appreciate an advocate there asking a bunch of questions from a logistical perspective, but they know that the advocate could provide pertinent information or prevent an error that could save the patient's life.

There is a high risk of infection in a hospital setting. When I was acting as a patient advocate, I sat for several days in an ICU room. I watched as people came in and out, pulling back the curtain each time. There were medical personnel, hospital staff, and visitors coming and going. There was a sink outside the curtain where doctors and nurses stopped to wash their hands and put on their clean gloves before coming in to examine the patient. Visitors, food service personnel, and housekeeping staff went from room to room touching the curtains of every patient and not washing their hands. Each time someone came in and pulled the curtain open and closed, I couldn't help but wonder what was lurking on that curtain, and subsequently on their hands or gloves.

According to the Centers for Disease Control, 5 to 10 percent of all patients get a healthcare-associated infection. That correlates to 1.7 million cases of infection caused by treatment and 99,000 deaths per year in the US. My point is that our traditional opinions about medical treatment and hospitals aren't always the best path for each of us. Remain informed, and don't be afraid to advocate for your health and treatment when necessary.

## The Pitfalls of Electronic Medical Records (EMRs)

The benefit of medical records is that a patient's records are accessible in a large network and can aid other doctors or hospitals in reviewing records and expediting care. This could potentially save your life. If you were in an accident and taken to a random hospital unconscious, staff could theoretically look you up and find out what conditions, allergies, or other health problems you have and medications you are on.

In 2014, the US government made it a requirement for medical practices to get on board with electronic medical records (EMRs) and penalized them in the form of reduced Medicare reimbursements for not doing it. They also subsidized medical practices in getting set up to implement EMRs in exchange for getting permanent access to their patients' medical records—your records.

I have a number of issues with this system from a logistical perspective as a medical assistant, from a patient perspective, and from an ethical perspective. First of all, the privacy paperwork you are likely required to sign does not protect you. It protects the "establishment." Anyone on the system or anyone they deem worthy of having your medical records can access your information, while you are limited in what you are able to see from your electronic records.

You are consenting to any "future" changes that are made to these policies without knowing what those changes might entail.

The EMR system was also intended to eliminate physical paperwork. I have found it generates just as much paper as the old paper system. The response is that an EMR can cause bias for a patient seeking a second opinion. I went to a GI doctor for a second opinion. The doctor came into the treatment room looking over a report that he had pulled off the system from another facility. I never authorized him to get the records and did not want his opinion to be biased before he even listened to me. In many cases a doctor will respect and accept the opinion of a colleague that is documented in the system unless they grossly disagree.

There are a number of different EMR systems, and they are not compatible. If you have treatment or testing at a facility that is on one EMR system, it will not show up on a different system. Medical offices, testing centers, and hospitals in the same community can be on separate systems.

Anything you say during a visit or anything that is documented about you can become part of your permanent record. Your personal information can be added to a government database and you could be "studied" without your knowledge or consent. There is no guarantee that your records are secure. While there are measures in place to protect the information, it is only as safe as anything can be that is stored in the Cloud. Anything can be hacked. Many practices outsource the scanning of all your records from a paper system to an electronic database, further jeopardizing the security of your personal information.

## The Future of Medicine

Medicine is becoming more regulated, and the mandates are driving some doctors out of the system. The drug companies are making the guidelines that the medical institutions must follow. They must adhere to the protocols to get reimbursed from insurance companies and to protect their license.

It is frustrating for those in the medical field because it limits, or in some cases prohibits, the doctor or nurse from making judgment calls. Judgment calls from experienced medical professionals have saved countless lives. Any deviation from the protocol will need to be justified, documented, and defended. In some cases it is not worth it for a professional to follow their gut instincts on a patient that they may have known for many years. Individualized care will be lost over time with this new system.

In the twenty-first century, thinking outside of the box is critical to healing. We are very unique creatures, and we are being forced into a cookie-cutter model. The new medical model does not leave the patient or the practitioner with many choices unless you stand up for what you believe.

Many hospitals are adopting a hospitalist approach where only their staff can treat you. In the past, your doctor may have had hospital rights to come into the hospital to monitor and treat you, order tests, and adjust drugs. Your doctor may not be able to see you in the hospital in this new environment.

**So . . . What Can You Do?**

My intention is not to steer you away from conventional medicine. It is to help you see that there are flaws in the system and help you find a better way. It is to get you thinking outside the box. Chances are, that is where you will find the answers to help you heal from any chronic illness you may have developed. The term "standard of care" is inaccurate. We are all unique and distinctive. We are not standardized. So our medical treatment and choices should not be either.

Encourage your doctor to reduce your medications. Whenever a medication or a procedure is ordered, ask why it is necessary and what are the risks or side effects. Also ask about the benefits. How successful is the medication? You can always ask your doctor if he or she would do this treatment if they were in your situation. Be your own advocate. Ask if there is a less invasive treatment. Ask how long you will need to be on the medication and what the long-term risks are. Be sure to tell your doctor if you experience any side effects from the medication.

Periodically ask your doctors to review your medications and see if there is something that can be eliminated. If you are going to be on the medication for an extended period, ask if it is known to deplete any nutrient in your body that you can supplement. If you chose to supplement, take a high-quality product, not something from a big-box store because products from these stores generally contain synthetic ingredients.

Do not blindly accept everything your doctor suggests. He or she must follow protocols. Understand that they may be insulted if you don't agree with them. They may need to document that you are refusing a certain treatment in order to protect themselves from liability. I have been asked to sign something stating that I was refusing a specific treatment. That is fine because they have the same right to protect themselves as I do. Conduct your own research. You are there to seek options. You are not there to discredit them nor to blindly accept everything they recommend. A good doctor will level with you and respect your choices. They may not agree with you. They may get on board with your choices because they need to practice within the scope of their license and follow the guidelines that they have been taught. They may not understand your position, and that is okay. It is not their journey, it is yours. It is your health, not theirs, and of course, it is your life, not theirs.

Guidelines change all the time. No one has all the answers. When I was having my children, it seemed every couple of years they were changing the guidelines on whether babies should sleep on their stomach or their back. I remember thinking I had put my previous baby at risk by "doing it wrong." We shouldn't beat ourselves up for choices we have made in the past when the choice was made with the best of intentions with the information we knew to be true at the time. We try so hard to do the right thing, but who defines what is right? They are simply opinions backed by some research or observations, and sometimes it is determined by someone with a special interest in you following that guideline.

Now, more than ever, we must take our power back. We don't have to be rebellious. We simply need to learn the facts and understand our options. You don't have to spend a ton of time doing extensive research. Find someone you trust who can offer you opinions. Do basic research on the topics that are most important to you. Form your own opinion. I am not asking you to have blind faith in everything I say. I speak my truth based on my experiences and insights. I am asking you to be cautious about having faith in any organization or industry that gains financially from what they are telling you.

Doctors do not know everything. They are human. They are also sometimes wrong. They are doing the best they can. They do not know your body better than you do.

Treat the underlying cause of the problem medically or holistically. Do not rely on long-term use of pharmaceutical drugs to manage an illness. Long-term use can cause more problems than it solves. You want to engage your doctors to prevent a health crisis and in the event of an accident or emergency. Listen to your inner wisdom and trust your gut. If something doesn't feel right to you, don't accept it.

As a patient, here are some things you can do to advocate for your sustained health and review treatment options before making a decision:

- *When you seek help from your doctor for a symptom, let your doctor know that you want to find and address the cause of the problem.*
- *Encourage your doctor to reduce your medications under their supervision.*
- *If you are put on a new drug, ask your doctor what lifestyle changes you can make to correct any behavior that may have led to the need for this medication. Ask how long you will need to stay on the drug. Always start at the lowest dose the doctor will allow.*
- *Be sure to keep a list of your current medications on your phone or in your wallet.*
- *Do your own research.*
- *Ask questions. Know the risks and benefits.*
- *Trust your gut instincts.*
- *Know that you have the right to opt out of having your records reported in certain databases. Review the privacy policy for your doctor's office or hospital, and inform the clerical staff when you fill out your*

*paperwork.*

- *Always have an advocate with you if you need to be hospitalized.*
- *Pack some healthy food for a hospital stay, or arrange for someone to bring you healthy food, filtered water, and snacks of fruit and raw vegetables. Most people are willing to help if you ask. Be sure to let the nurse or doctor know in case there is any medical reason to restrict what you eat.*
- *Focus your mind on the outcome you want instead of on the problem at hand.*
- *Keep your body healthy to prevent the need for medical intervention.*

Implementing even a few of these helpful tips and resources will almost certainly shift your perspective and better position you to make informed and knowledgeable decisions. In the end, we only have one body, one mind, and one life. This chapter should help provide you with the crucial tools to make the most of it.

## The Happiness Quotient

One of my jobs involves gathering patient intake information in a medical practice. Each patient is required to answer the question, "Are you depressed?" It is disturbing to me that so many people answer "yes" to this question. How is it possible that we accept this? How can so many people be struggling to enjoy their life? Why is it that so many people feel hopeless and even helpless to improve their experience? What can be done to truly change this? I don't believe medication is the answer. As humanity and as a profession, how can we contribute to finding a better way to help people? The suggestions I offer will help people find health and happiness in their lives, but not everyone is capable or has the capacity to take responsibility for their happiness.

Life is moving so quickly. It is sometimes impossible to keep up with the pace. It is causing a lot of anxiety for people, especially as they age. As they get into a state of fear, they lose the ability to stay in the present moment and are unable to experience joy. Many people are in a victim mindset. We have very little power when we feel we are a victim of our circumstances. Many people don't realize they have options, have been conditioned to believe they are powerless, have resigned themselves to their current state, and have become content with the fact that they have no zest for life.

For those of us who have the capacity, we must first heal our own lives. As each of us takes responsibility for our health and happiness and raises our vibration, we contribute to the collective vibration of the planet. Once we achieve a higher level of joy and vitality, we can be of service to others.

Instead of asking patients if they are depressed, shouldn't we be asking, "Are you happy?" If not, why not?

Which areas of your life or health are not working for you? What would you need to be happy and healthy? How can we help you get there? How can we get these people thinking about their capacity to be proactive about their health and happiness? How can we get them to focus on what they want? Shouldn't we be measuring health and happiness instead of depression and disease?

### *How Can You Raise Your Happiness Quotient?*

Start by taking a moment to assess your life and ask yourself what it would take to make your life better. Think outside the box. What would truly make you happy? What do you need more of in your life? What do you need less of? What would your life look like if you were happier and had more robust health? What small step can you take to get even a little bit closer to realizing more health and happiness? As you read on, you will gain insight as to what those steps might be.

# Chapter 4

## The Hidden Toxins on Your Table

Your body must make decisions about each and every thing you ingest. It decides if you are supplying nutrients that need to be extracted and assimilated or if you have eaten something that needs to be detoxified. Sadly, many components of our food and water are toxic. We are not designed to digest molecules that our bodies can't recognize as coming from nature. True health is about balance and harmony in the body. There are many things that disrupt the body's natural state of harmony.

Many of us mistakenly believe the industries regulating our food are looking out for our best interests. In working with clients over almost two decades, I have found many toxic ingredients that have caused distress for those people and animals. While all of these ingredients are generally recognized as "safe," there are growing concerns about their actual safety. Whether you realize you are exposing yourself to harmful substances or not, as you increase your toxic load, damage is being done.

Food sensitivities and dietary and environmental toxins create physiological as well as energetic disruptions in your body. You may not realize that you are exposing yourself to toxins on a daily basis. If you are eating a standard convenience diet, you are probably eating many toxins. The good news is that it is never too late to clean up your diet and your surroundings.

My intention in sharing the grim truths about the toxicity of the modern diet is not to take the pleasure out of your eating experience. It is to empower you with the knowledge you need to make the best choices so that you can optimize your health and possibly even reverse disease. You can live a healthy and bountiful life while eating delicious and nutrient-rich food.

Junk food is an oxymoron. You eat food or you eat junk. You can pay up front for healthier, more nutrient-rich food, or pay the price later to undo the damage done by less conscientious products. Knowledge is power. The most important thing we can do for ourselves is to feed our bodies and minds healthfully and to make informed, conscious decisions about what we are eating. That is the purpose of this chapter.

The fate of our food supply is in our hands. As consumers, we maintain tremendous power to change the way our food is grown and manufactured. Food manufacturers listen. When they see trends in the market, they respond to them. In the early 2000s, it was hard to find the organic section in a grocery store. It was often a dusty shelf with a small selection of packaged goods that looked and tasted rather boring. Some stores carried a small selection of organic produce and refrigerated products that often looked wilted and were at the end of their shelf life. I considered myself at the forefront of the non-GMO and organic food movement. I would buy that dusty box of organic cereal in hopes that the store would continue to offer it. Today, there are large sections of produce and packaged organic food in beautiful displays in predominant locations in most grocery stores. Many manufacturers are removing artificial food dyes, GMOs, and preservatives from their products because of trends in consumer-buying habits. They are listening and responding to our requests and consumer practices. It is no coincidence.

## Genetically Modified Organisms (GMOs)

I have not been without health challenges. I needed to go through those challenges so I could learn why I was here. Years ago when I was struggling with a mystery illness, I was diagnosed with gastroesophageal reflux (GERD), stomach ulcers, esophageal ulcers, and duodenal ulcers. I saw several doctors and gastroenterology specialists. Everyone wanted to put me on drugs. I knew my body was in serious distress, and it was not going to get better unless something changed. It needed to change fast because disease was setting in. It was painful and scary. The doctors agreed I had too much stomach acid and that I needed to take drugs for the ulcers and to reduce the acid. I did not believe my body was malfunctioning and producing too much acid. I knew there was a root cause. I just didn't know what it was.

I agreed to start the drugs until I could figure out the

cause. I knew that the acid-reducing drug, a proton pump inhibitor, could cause havoc on my body if I took it for months on end. In fact, it could permanently alter my body's ability to produce stomach acid, which is essential for digestion. I researched the drug and knew it would not be safe for me in the long term. Time was of the essence. During the first week on the drugs, I found the pain was reduced significantly, but I developed headaches and severe problems digesting my food. I believed my diet was healthy, but my food was quickly passing through my body undigested. This horrified me. The scientist in me knew if my food was completely undigested, I would not be able to assimilate any nutrients and my health would suffer.

The doctors wanted me on these drugs to prevent harm, but the drugs were causing harm. Without the drugs, I would risk perforating my stomach, esophagus, or colon in the short term, any of which could be life threatening. Without the drugs, I would risk further disease, including cancer of any of those areas over the long term. With the drugs short term, I would face acute distress in the form of headaches, food passing undigested, and nutritional deficiencies. These options were unacceptable.

My doctors kept sending me for endoscopies and colonoscopies, where they took biopsies. I felt these tests were damaging my body. I would bleed for days after the biopsies and knew that any of these biopsy sites could tear. I even questioned my doctor about whether all the biopsies were necessary. Before the last endoscopy, I wrote all over the form that I did not give them permission to take biopsies and would only consent to the test to see visually the state of my insides. I told the anesthesiologist and doctor this before they put me under. After the test, I felt a lot more discomfort and didn't understand why until I went for the follow-up a week later and in the report they said all eight biopsies were benign. I was furious that the doctor took the biopsies against my will while I was sedated. I felt violated and betrayed. I decided that I would not go back for any more of these tests.

By this time I had been doing food-sensitivity screening as part of my holistic coaching business. It was not uncommon to see trends where more people would start testing sensitive to something such as gluten, dairy, food dyes, or chemical preservatives. Suddenly, I started seeing a large percentage of clients who were testing sensitive to certain types of food at rates that were surprising to me. This food included corn and soy and, to a lesser extent, sugar and canola. I was getting feedback that their symptoms were improving or had completely resolved after eliminating this food. Sometimes after a client removed an offending food from their diet and noticed an improvement in their overall well-being or reduction in symptoms, I had them reintroduce the food a few weeks later and pay close attention to how their body responded. If that food is responsible for that specific symptom, I would expect that symptom to come back. In almost every case, the symptoms resolved after eliminating the food and returned after reintroducing the food.

This intrigued me, and I began searching for common factors and reasons why this food was suddenly causing so many problems. I was shocked by my findings. Several years earlier, this food had been genetically engineered and the new versions of it had quietly entered our food supply unannounced and virtually untested. The Internet was new to me at this time, and information was rather limited. However, I researched everything I could find about this food. It certainly made sense to me that this process could wreak havoc on our bodies. I believed the trend I was seeing in my clients was related to this engineering of our food. Essentially it just took several years for people's bodies to start showing the damage in the form of symptoms.

While I did not notice any acute symptoms when I consumed this food, I began to question if this newly engineered food could be causing my own health crisis. Could it be this simple? I began to carefully eliminate these GMOs from my diet. At the same time, I began weaning myself off the medications because of the side effects. I expected the heartburn, ulcers, and GERD to get worse as I weaned from the drugs. Much to my surprise, I felt better. After just two weeks of eliminating this food, I was completely off the drugs and I felt good.

Many medications must be weaned off under a doctor's supervision. I am not advocating that you stop your medications or go against your doctor's orders. These were my choices, and they were right for me at the time. I take responsibility for that decision. That was fifteen years ago at the time of this writing, and to this day when I eat GMOs I get heartburn. I believe that GMOs are devastating to our health and our environment. They are having a major impact on public health.

In my experience in helping people clean up their lives and their diets, I find GMOs are one of the worst dietary offenders that are making people sick. I scientifically and morally oppose the use of GMOs. Most prepared food today contain them. Currently, they are not required to be labeled. When I teach workshops, I ask participants if they eat GMOs. Most people say no. The truth is if you don't work hard to avoid them, you are eating them.

Food derived from these practices can destroy the human body's microbiome, which can cause us to be chronically inflamed and nutritionally depleted. We must understand that advancements in food science, crop science, and genetic modification won't improve upon nature. Don't eat things that don't come from nature or in a form that nature did not intend. If an apple doesn't rot, it is not good for you. Do not be fooled into thinking this science is simply improving upon nature. Each step your food takes away from its natural state is putting you a step closer to a state of dis-ease.

GMO crops that are herbicide tolerant are able to withstand a huge amount of herbicide, such as glyphosate. Since GMOs have been approved, the amount of these herbicides applied to food crops has increased exponentially. University of California San Diego School of Medicine researchers estimate human exposure to glyphosate has increased approximately 500 percent. These herbicides have been found in our drinking water, air, blood, and vital organs. They have been linked to a variety of illnesses including cancers and nonalcoholic fatty liver disease. Glyphosate is a known carcinogen, and it can penetrate the blood-brain barrier.

Some weeds have become resistant to these herbicides, which has led biotechnology companies to develop seeds that will grow plants that are resistant to even more toxic herbicides such as 2,4-D, a component of Agent Orange.

At the time of the writing of this book, there are nine GMO crops that are allowed in the US. Additional crops have been approved and may enter the market. If you live in another country, I urge you to investigate which GMO food is approved for planting, selling, and importing in your country. For example, GMO Salmon is approved in Canada. Since GMOs are not required to be labeled, to avoid GMOs you should not buy products with these ingredients unless they are organic or have the "NON-GMO Project Verified" label.

The GMO crops are:

- *Corn*
- *Soy*
- *Canola*
- *Cottonseed*
- *Zucchini*
- *Yellow crooked neck squash*
- *Hawaiian papaya*
- *Sugar beets*
- *Alfalfa*

Many more GMO seeds are awaiting approval. The only way to stop more of this food from getting approved and entering the food chain is to speak up before it gets approved. Once a GMO crop is planted, it is almost impossible to contain or recall it once the pollen has spread and possibly even cross-pollinated other crops. I am constantly sending letters to my politicians and encouraging others to do so as well. It is not that difficult, and once you do it for the first time, it becomes quick and easy. Corporations, industries, and the government will often take away our rights unless we work to protect them.

Many people feel GMOs are the result of corporate greed and have no place in our diets or our environment. I believe God has created each plant in nature to a level of perfection that we will never fully understand, and it is not likely that we can improve upon nature. If the biotech companies that are selling GMO seed for our food supply really believe they are superior and are not harming us, they should be proud to support manufacturers to label their products as containing GMOs. Instead they have spent billions of dollars lobbying and fighting GMO labeling.

As an activist, I fought for GMO labeling. There was a time when industries told us they could not label products that contained GMOs because it would ultimately cost too much money and would drive up the price of food. That was simply not true. Companies did not want to label GMOs. They were afraid of losing market share if consumers knew their food products contained GMO ingredients. In reality, companies are constantly changing their labels for various reasons including special promotions and to raise awareness of the causes they support. Many companies have even changed their labels to promote that their product is "NON-GMO Project Verified." For many companies, this label has increased sales.

Companies are beginning to voluntarily remove food dyes, preservatives, GMOs, and stop using hormones and antibiotics on their animals. It is a start. I realized long ago as an activist for cleaner food that the government would not likely mandate changes. There are politics to consider and the interests of very powerful companies. Knowledge is key to protecting yourself. You can find resources to stay up to date on GMOs on my website, www.TapintoBalance.com.

## Food Dyes

I consider all artificial food dyes to be toxic. Artificial food dyes are derived from compounds such as petroleum and coal tars. Many studies have shown food dyes to be neurotoxins, and some countries have banned certain dyes. I have seen numerous cases where symptoms of irritability, hyperactivity, inability to focus, learning disabilities, rashes, hives, headaches, and even dyslexia have completely resolved when dyes have been eliminated. In my personal experience, I have seen the most problems with red dye #40, yellow dye #5, and yellow dye #6. Yellow #5 is also known as tartrazine.

To eliminate food dyes, educate yourself and carefully read the ingredient labels, looking for the words *yellow*, *blue*, *red*, or *artificial color*.

Here are some food and products that may contain artificial dyes and some suggestions for alternatives:

- *Many breakfast cereals, even if they are not the sweet, colorful varieties*
- *Pickles*
- *Salmon that is farm-raised often is fed red dye. Wild salmon is a better choice.*
- *Chickens are often fed tartrazine to make their egg yolks more yellow. Buy eggs from responsible companies. Buy only eggs from chicken or fowl that are cage free, that aren't fed hormones or antibiotics. Consider buying organic eggs.*

- *Candy*
- *Gelatin desserts*
- *Chewing gum*
- *Cake mixes*
- *Fruit snacks. Don't confuse "natural" or "made with real fruit juice" claims with fruit snacks that are truly made from fruit. While they may contain real fruit or fruit juice, the former are often made of corn syrup, gelatin, artificial flavors, and food dyes.*
- *Yellow American cheese. White cheeses or other naturally colored cheeses make a good alternative. Note that some contain hormones and antibiotics. Some lower-cost shredded cheeses on the market are not actually cheese. Read the packaging.*
- *Beverages such as sports drinks, juices, lemonade, flavored teas, and soda.*
- *Medications, both over-the-counter and prescription. Seek dye-free alternatives.*
- *Colors derived from fruits or vegetables are the best option.*

## Chemical Additives

Food additives are a multibillion-dollar industry. Additives can extend shelf life, inhibit microbial growth, and improve taste, appearance, or texture.

Many food additives that have been approved as safe for food use have later been found to be toxic. I am unaware of any studies that look at the toxicity of different combinations of food additives. Be especially cautious about eating food products with multiple chemicals in them. It is left for the manufacturers to determine if the additive is safe. This is a potential conflict of interest because the manufacturer has a lot to gain if the additive is found safe and a lot to lose if it is found to be unsafe or toxic.

It is interesting that some countries can determine that an additive is toxic, ban it from use in food, and refuse to import products with that ingredient from other countries. Other countries may consider that same ingredient to be safe and may use it extensively in food products, even in products consumed primarily by babies and children.

Many people have sensitivities or experience reactions to preservatives, such as headaches, rashes, digestive upset, dizziness, or irritability.

Some additives to avoid:

- *Aluminum or alum*
- *Butylated hydroxyanisole (BHA)*
- *Butylated hydroxytoluene (BHT)*
- *Propylene glycol*
- *Sulfites*
- *Sulfur dioxide*
- *Guar gum*
- *Methylene chloride (used to decaffeinate coffee)*
- *Monopotassium glutamate*

- *Monosodium glutamate (MSG)*
- *Nitrates*
- *Nitrites*
- *Polysorbate*
- *Tertiary butylhydroquinone (TBHQ)*

You have the right to ask an employee of a restaurant, deli, or bakery to see the ingredient list for any food they sell. Most franchises will list their ingredients on their website under nutrition information or allergy information. I urge anyone eating fast food to look at the ingredients before eating another bite.

I opt for a family-owned restaurant over large chain restaurants. In many cases, the food is prepared on site, fresher, and less processed. There is no reason to add chemicals to fresh food, so the easiest way to avoid chemicals is to eat fresh whole food and prepare food yourself. Read the ingredient list on the packaging of any prepared or convenience food.

## Sweeteners

While all sugars have deleterious effects on the body, artificial sweeteners are of particular concern. They are used in food and beverages such as chewing gums, sports drinks, yogurt, flavored water, and food labeled as sugar-free, low-calorie, low-carbohydrate, and low-sugar. You will also find them in packets on restaurant tables.

Artificial and "natural" sweeteners to avoid include:

- *Acesulfame-K (acesulfame potassium)*
- *Aspartame*
- *Sucralose*
- *Saccharin*
- *Corn syrup*
- *High fructose corn syrup*
- *Refined white sugar*

White sugar is often made from a combination of beet sugar, which is often a GMO, and cane sugar. It can be heavily processed and bleached. While all sugar is refined, in my opinion, raw, organic turbinado, or unbleached cane sugar, is best. Honey, molasses, and date sugar are good options. Stevia and xylitol are acceptable low-calorie options and should be used in moderation as both are often heavily processed.

## Pesticides

Pesticide use around the world has dramatically increased over the past few decades. We can't see the pesticides and toxins on our food, but chronic exposure spells chronic disease. It is hard to find commercially grown food that is not contaminated. Some pesticides persist in the soil, and many accumulate in the food chain and in our bodies. Even small-term exposure or ingestion over time can have devastating effects on our health.

Conventionally grown food that often contains high levels of pesticide residue are:

- *Corn*
- *Wheat*
- *Peanuts*
- *Strawberries*
- *Apples*
- *Spinach*
- *Grapes*
- *Peaches*
- *Potatoes*

The Environmental Working Group is a sound resource for identifying toxic food and products to avoid as well as food and products that are safe. They study and publish an annual "Dirty Dozen" and a "Clean 15" list for produce. Watch for their list each year to stay current. Visit my website, www.TapintoBalance.com for links to helpful resources.

To reduce the amount of pesticides you consume, buy organic versions of this food and if possible, grow your own.

**Deceptive Facts**

It is refreshing that conscientious consumers have shifted the market. Several decades ago, everything in the supermarket was fairly clean. This changed after years of technology, pesticide use, genetic engineering, adding chemical preservatives, and processing practices were implemented to prolong shelf life. It seemed like a great idea to the companies, but consumers had little knowledge of what was happening to their food supply.

Industries are wise to what some consumers are eliminating and will actually mislead you. The labels that we count on are deceptive.

Sometimes a company will swap out one preservative for another. The front of the label boasts that they no longer have a specific toxic ingredient in the product, but what they don't advertise on the front of the package is that they have replaced that toxic chemical preservative with a different one. The consumer gets a false sense of security. Read your labels carefully, and strive to obtain as much information as you can.

Nutrition facts can be deceptive simply by altering the serving size. I'm not here to make the argument that trans fats are dangerous and can impair your health and lead to heart disease. This fact is pretty universally accepted, and most people work to avoid it. Trans fat is required to be on the nutrition label. Serving size is key in the case of trans fats, and to illustrate my point, in the following example I will use cookies that are labeled as containing "0 grams of trans fat." Assume a serving size of two cookies. Each cookie contains 0.2 grams of trans fat. For a serving size of two cookies, there will be 0.4 grams of trans fat. There are several ways that rounding numbers is allowed. In this case, 0.4 can be rounded down to 0. It is misleading because you believe the product contains NO trans fats and the front label on the product boasts that it contains "0 grams of trans fat." Yet if you eat four of these cookies, you have just consumed nearly one gram of trans fat without even knowing it.

Companies are aware that consumers are beginning to avoid certain ingredients. I have seen products with large banners across the front label that advertise the product is made without high fructose corn syrup. Upon turning the product around, you may find one of the top ingredients is corn syrup. I have also seen products that boast no corn syrup in the product, yet high fructose corn syrup is one of the main ingredients.

Many consumers now avoid aspartame. Interestingly, a name change was approved to use the name AminoSweet to rebrand aspartame. This is misleading because it sounds a little healthier, and those who are avoiding aspartame may not know they are still consuming it under a different name. It seems unreasonable that companies would not simply replace the sweetener with a healthier choice.

A label claim that a product is "natural" or "all-natural" really means nothing. This claim looks good to consumers and gives us a false sense of security about the integrity of the product. Read the ingredient list carefully, and you will often find some questionable ingredients.

Companies are not required by law to put an ingredient

on the label if they do not add it to the product. An example of this would be monosodium glutamate (MSG). If a company adds a raw material to a formula that contains MSG, but they do not add MSG as part of their recipe, they do not have to put MSG on the ingredient list.

To illustrate, Company A makes soup bouillon and they add MSG to that product. They provide this raw material to Company B, which makes soup and produces it in a canned version to sell directly to consumers and supplies it to restaurants. As long as Company B does not add additional MSG to their recipe, they do not have to list MSG on the ingredient list of their finished soup product. Therefore, a consumer in the supermarket reads the label on the can and is happy to see that it does not contain MSG. Likewise, when a person asks a server in a restaurant if their soup has MSG, the server checks with the chef and determines the soup does not contain it. In either scenario, the consumer unknowingly gets MSG.

In most cases, companies want to sell their product at the lowest cost. They use marketing strategies on the label that best sell the product. It is legal, but if you do not understand these practices, you may be deceived.

## Take a Toxin Inventory

Ask yourself where you are getting toxins in your diet. Take an inventory of the food you eat regularly. Read the labels and check for any ingredients mentioned in this chapter.

You may be surprised to find toxic ingredients in your food even if you think you are eating a healthy diet. To point out some sources of hidden toxicity, I provide an example of a healthy choice lunch. If your meal consists of only a large salad full of raw veggies, you could be eating toxins. For instance, there may be sliced GMO zucchini or yellow squash on the salad, or the dressing many contain GMO sugar, GMO corn sweeteners such as corn syrup or high fructose corn syrup, and GMO vegetable oil such as canola or soybean oil. Commercial salad dressings often contain chemical preservatives such as monosodium glutamate. The vegetables may also contain pesticides that have been taken up by the roots of the plants. Think about how carnations are often dyed by simply adding a couple of drops of food coloring to their water. The food coloring is taken up by the cut flower via the stems from the dyed water supply. There is no way to wash off the dye that is within the stems or flowers. No amount of washing will remove what is inside the plant. Vegetables are sometimes commercially washed with chemical products as well. Residues often remain on the produce. Other potentially toxic ingredients may be negatively affecting you if you add croutons, cheese, or processed luncheon meat to your salad. We won't go through all of them in this text.

All of these toxins have consequences when consumed over time. Most people will not fall sick from eating the salad just mentioned. Because toxins accumulate in the body, every time you can make a better choice, your body will be spared further damage, is better equipped to detoxify, and can utilize the nutrients in the food to support your health.

Here are tips to help you reduce your toxic load:

- *Avoid GMO ingredients.*
- *Avoid food dyes.*
- *Avoid chemical additives.*
- *Avoid artificial sweeteners.*
- *Select food in its most natural state.*
- *Limit the amount of food you eat that contains chemical ingredients.*
- *Cook your own meals so you know what you are eating.*
- *Remember, you have the right to ask storekeepers or restaurant employees about food ingredients.*
- *While eating out, you can special order your food to be prepared in a safer way or to omit ingredients that pose a risk.*
- *Buy organic when you can.*
- *Buy food that is in season and grown locally.*
- *Plant a garden or grow your favorite produce in containers.*
- *Grow your own herbs to healthfully enhance the flavor of your food.*

## Your Body Will Thank You

Finding a good balance for yourself will help you feel better and enjoy life as well. You don't want to get in the practice of depriving yourself and being so strict that you feel you are on a diet all of the time.

Start by making informed choices and eating better. Your taste buds adapt and your body will thank you by restoring your health, increasing your energy, and producing a feeling of well-being. Eat food in its most natural form or that has ingredients you recognize as being something you might have in your kitchen. If you can't picture it or pronounce it, don't eat it. Eat food that is in season and grown locally when you can. Frequent your local farmers market.

It is amazing how quickly your body will recognize the value in what you are eating and begin to love the taste of superhealthy food. It will also begin to dislike the "junk" food that once pleased you. I remember when I started drinking green juice. The first sip tasted horrible, and I continued to drink it anyway because I knew it had great benefits. The second drink was a bit more palatable and tasted like peas. As my body started to recognize the value in it, I started to like it. Within a few days, I began to crave it. Now I love it. The same may happen for you. As you clean up your diet, you will find your body loves the healthier food. You will learn to enjoy the taste, feel satisfied more quickly, and experience a new sense of vibrancy.

# Chapter 5

## The Trouble with Technology: When Smart Is Not So Smart

In September of 2015, I received a notice stating that my power company had installed a smart meter on my house. I was not happy about this, because I knew the meter gave the power company personal customer usage data to sell to marketing companies. I felt it was more an issue of data mining and an invasion of privacy than a threat to my personal health. I had some concerns though. At the time, I had a meter that measures extremely low-frequency (ELF) electromagnetic fields (EMFs). I placed my EMF meter close to the smart meter to see what type of measurements I might find. The readings were extremely high near the smart meter, which is also next to the main power supply coming into the house. Away from the meter, the readings were low. I also measured the inside of the house, since the adjacent room is my son's bedroom. Everything appeared fine as long as it was not within about five feet of the meter.

Soon after, I began to notice that I was having trouble sleeping. I run on less sleep than most people because I am usually feverishly working on a book or some research that has me pretty well consumed. This was different. I was tired but could not sleep. If I did fall asleep, I would awaken an hour later and was wide awake. I dismissed any correlation between this problem and the smart meter because the readings were low and I was on the opposite side of the house. I went on a couple of wild goose chases for answers but never could definitively figure it out. I started experiencing spikes in blood pressure and very high resting pulse rates. I had an electrocardiogram and an echocardiogram to rule out any heart condition.

I saw several doctors over the next year. At this point, I was only getting two to three hours of sleep per day. I was exhausted and began to have problems focusing and functioning. One doctor attributed this to anxiety. That didn't make sense. I am more at peace than most people I know, and I know how to release my stress. I did not believe it was an anxiety issue. My labs were all out of range, but nothing jumped out as the specific cause of these issues. Another doctor suggested hyperthyroidism, which matched my symptoms. Another specialist said my thyroid was switching between hypoactive and hyperactive, but did not feel my thyroid was bad enough to treat. I developed a large, painful lymphatic tumor and some swollen lymph nodes. My lymphocytes were three times the normal level. I developed high fevers at night with chills, sweating, and violent shivering for six weeks. Another doctor tried to convince me that the insomnia was due to menopause and that the night fevers were hot flashes. I knew this was not the case. My body temperature registered 101 - 102°F at night and 97 - 98°F in the morning. I was shivering and would sweat when I broke the fever. My health continued to deteriorate. The root cause was never determined.

I knew for certain that I did not want to seek any further traditional medical treatment and did not want to start biopsying and treating any "disease." I did not want to limit myself to chasing and treating the symptoms. I decided I did not want to seek a diagnosis. By the end of 2016, I knew I was seriously ill, and I did not want to give the illness any power by labeling it. It would not serve me or my family to label it. I did not want the stigma, sympathy, or worries associated with it. I only wanted to find the cause and eliminate it so I could work on restoring my health.

I knew this experience was a necessary part of my spiritual journey. I had to put this book on hold because I was too sick to function. I had severe fatigue, exhaustion, and could not think clearly. My heart raced and I had shortness of breath. I forced myself to eat organic applesauce each day because it was the only food that did not make me feel nauseous. I closed the files of this book and put them away for almost six months. Other than keeping several commitments per week, I spent four months in bed. I knew only one thing for certain, and that was that my life was writing a chapter of this book. I knew at a very deep level that I had to live through this long enough to write about it, and if I didn't, I had made arrangements to ensure the book would get done without me. I didn't know what this chapter would be about and I had assumed it would be about exit points. Exit points are what I call those times in our lives when we are offered the opportunity to leave this life at a soul level to move on to something else.

I could not figure out what was causing this or what I needed to do to heal. I was feeling a bit defeated because nothing was working. I was losing hope that I would be able to figure this out, and I knew there was a cause that I was missing. If this illness was going to progress, I did not want to opt for surgery or drug treatments. At a core level, I did not believe either of those options would serve me. My body rejected any supplements. I could not assimilate nutrients, and my body was not detoxifying. I felt like I was being poisoned. My life force was slipping away. I surrendered to the possibility that this might be my fate.

While I did turn to traditional medicine to get help in finding the cause of my symptoms, doctors were unable to come up with any answers that satisfied me. I feel it is necessary to share my journey to provide you an understanding of how I came through it and what I have learned about the cause of this illness.

## Seeking Holistic Help

I felt my only hope was to turn to my dear friend and naturopath for help. We agreed that a diagnosis would not serve me. He indicated it was too late for any supplements to aid in my recovery. He suggested I jump on my rebounder (mini-trampoline) for five minutes twice per day. I could only jump for about one minute. It was painful to jump, and my extreme fatigue and rapid pulse made it feel as if my eyes were going to pop out of my head. He also suggested that I use my chi machine. A chi machine is a mechanical device that shakes your body. The idea behind the rebounder and chi machine is to get your lymphatic fluid moving. I used the chi machine every day for a couple of weeks.

One day, the lymphatic tumor in my underarm was particularly painful as I shook on the chi machine. I began to feel very fearful about the tumor. Fear is a very destructive emotion, and I have listened to many great thought leaders speak on fear. I remembered a story shared by a woman who decided she did not want to hate and fight the cancer that was growing in her body. Instead, she loved her tumors and healed from cancer. It was a mindset adjustment that brought to mind a scenario where Mother Teresa refused to attend a war demonstration, but would happily join a peace rally. It was a matter of supporting the right side of the issue. Mother Teresa said that we need to find God and that He could not be found in noise and restlessness. She also said that our strength lies in small things. Through those thoughts, I realized what I must do. In that moment, I made the decision to love that tumor. I held my hand over it and sent it love with my intention. I thanked it for getting my attention, for causing me to slow down, teaching me to take better care of myself, and prompting me to look for the cause. I relaxed into the realization that I could stay in fear or transmute that into love. It was my choice how I reacted to this fear and pain. Obviously, love is very powerful and positive and more conducive to healing than fear. Three days later, the tumor was gone.

A few days after that, my friend passed from this life. He had facilitated more healing than anyone I know. He had a brilliant way of making light of serious conditions and turning them around quickly and inexpensively. He was the one I would send my toughest client cases to. The one I turned to if I couldn't figure something out. Life would never be quite the same. My sons reminded me that it was time for me to pick up the torch. I realized I needed to muster my strength and use my own advice. I had to think about what I would suggest for someone who came to me in this condition.

## The Shocking Realization

A couple weeks later as I was lying in bed thinking about all of this, I began to ask for answers. Why isn't anything helping? Is it too late for any nutrients to help? What does my body need? Why can't I figure this out? What am I missing? What do I need to know? I had been able to solve all of my health challenges in the past. There had to be a higher reason I was experiencing this. I began a conversation with God. *Is this my fate? Really? Why am I enduring all this if it is just to die?* There had to be more to it, more to do. I was open to being used in service and for a higher purpose, but I had to be able to make sense of it. I needed an answer. Then out of nowhere, I heard very clearly: "The smart meter."

My initial response was, "No way." I climbed out of my bed, where I had spent the majority of the last four months, and went downstairs to my computer to search "symptoms caused by smart meter exposure." As I began to read the results, I found that I had thirteen of the fifteen most commonly reported symptoms related to radiofrequency (RF) exposure.

I had never heard of anyone getting sick from smart meters or radiofrequency. I was shocked, angry, and relieved to have something to pursue. I felt my passion coming back. This was a moment of tremendous power. I realized the EMF meter I had used a year earlier to measure my smart meter when it was installed was not the proper type of meter. I started doing some research online and realized the only way I could investigate this was to order a radiofrequency meter and a body voltage meter. The meters arrived days later. As I opened the package, I knew these meters were either going to give me the answers I needed to validate my theory or leave me further defeated. I was hopeful, but I had no idea what I would find.

While I believe I have a pretty good understanding of the energetic field, in full disclosure, I know next to nothing about electricity or radiofrequencies. It was a learning curve for me to even operate these meters and understand what the readings meant. I took my first body voltage reading in the area of my home where I spent most of my time working over the past several years. My reading was 15.38 volts—an extremely high and shocking level. I thought I must have the scale wrong; it couldn't possibly be 15.38 volts. Upon further study, I realized the meter was correct. A level this high will halt many cellular functions. Tears of both terror and joy welled up in my eyes as I realized this invisible force was harming me. I had no idea how to protect myself or remedy the situation, but I now had the answer I needed and was ready to investigate. In that moment a friend texted me to ask how I was doing, and I quickly responded, "My smart meter is killing me." In that moment, I took back my power.

Over the next couple of weeks, I found that the radiofrequencies causing this health crisis were not only coming from my smart meter (the meter was a small part of the RF levels in my home), but that there were several major contributors in my house. These included my Wi-Fi router, the Wi-Fi enabled on the computers and devices in our house, my cell phone, my kids' cell phones, my microwave oven, my smart meter, my neighbors' Wi-Fi and smart meters, my three cordless phones, and the phone base station. The area of my home where I spent the majority of my waking hours is situated in the worst possible location in proximity to all of these sources.

I am still learning to manage this electrosensitivity. While our bodies may adapt to this technology over time, I do not believe it will happen in the near future. I will not resign myself to being exposed to radiofrequency to the extent that it continues to poison me. I am hopeful that the technology will change, that I can adequately shield myself to be able to live in harmony with technology, or my response will be to spend time in remote areas to limit my exposure and give my body time to heal. Either way, I will continue to find better ways to live with this technology until I find a solution.

This is not something traditional medicine knows anything about or has any idea how to treat. Nothing taught in medical school prepares doctors to identify this issue, and there is not a definitive test or marker in the blood that will lead to a diagnosis. It simply goes undiagnosed until it leads to chronic diseases that can be diagnosed and treated without finding the cause. I realized I was pretty much on my own to come to an understanding of what was going on and what I could do to fix it.

## Outsmarting Smart Devices

In sharing my story, I hope my wake-up call becomes your wake-up call. We can all take better care of ourselves as a result. I'm still learning about radiofrequencies and ways to shield them at the time of this writing. I do not know a lot about them, but do feel comfortable enough shouting it from the rooftop. It is too important of an issue to wait until I understand it all to warn people to take precautions. It is quite possible that it can take ten, twenty, even thirty years for people to develop illnesses from the cumulative effects of all the radiation we are exposed to. The truth is, in our modern society there is no way to be completely safe from radiofrequencies. As I learn more I will post information and resources on my website, www.TapintoBalance.com.

In reducing some of this radiation, I have recaptured my ability to think—enough so that I have been able to critically analyze my symptoms and all of my RF meter readings before and after taking action to reduce my exposure. I experience a hypersensitivity to radiofrequency exposure or radio wave sickness. Most people do not react as strongly as I do. I am essentially a canary in the coal mine. I have always felt one of my purposes is to experience things and to take on illnesses that I can figure out and later use to educate others. I have an insatiable curiosity to understand things. This is my nature. I feel confident in saying that radiofrequencies were killing me and they are harming many people. I believe they are the cause of many symptoms, mystery illnesses, and over time can lead or contribute to diseases such as diabetes, thyroid disorders, heart disease, Alzheimer's, lymphoma, and leukemia. I have found there are increasing numbers of people around the world who have an electromagnetic hypersensitivity (EHS). In fact, some countries recognize EHS as a disability.

According to Dietrich Klinghardt, MD, PhD, this electromagnetic pollution is an emerging health risk and even those who are not sensitive or experiencing symptoms are being harmed. Industry studies do not back this up and show very little effect on living organisms. In most cases, industry studies have found the only effect is electrostimulation and heating of body tissue when devices are held close to the body. I have found references to a couple of thousand independent studies that show the potential harm to the body that are not based on heating of tissue.

Dr. Klinghardt, a practicing physician in the US and Germany specializing in chronic illness, states that manmade electromagnetic frequencies in the high-frequency range are devastating to our health. These frequencies alter our brain proteins, which affect virtually all cellular functions. In his medical practices, he sees a number of symptoms and illnesses related to radiofrequency exposure; these include insomnia, depression, neurological symptoms such as tingling, numbness, and vibrations in the body, muscle aches, fatigue, headaches, learning disabilities, and autism. He has seen devastating consequences from smart meters and says they pose one of the most significant threats to our health. Dr. Klinghardt has also found that radiation is concentrated in the womb and that pregnant women need to take precautionary measures to protect themselves and their unborn babies.

The way I understand it is that when our bodies are in contact with RF radiation, it is absorbed by our skin. These manmade frequencies are irritating to the skin and cause the cells to secrete stress hormones and other factors that circulate through our bodies. When the voltage in our bodies is high enough, it essentially makes our cell membranes harden or leak to the extent that our cells cannot properly carry out their normal functions. The chemical processes that normally occur at a cellular level are suppressed. Our cellular metabolism becomes disrupted. An imbalance occurs in the calcium levels in and around our cells. Some things that may occur as a result are that our normal hormonal cycles can be disrupted, which also cause sleep disturbances. We may have increases in free radical damage and oxidative stress. In addition, we may experience mitochondrial dysfunction affecting our energy levels, inflammatory processes being initiated, brain proteins being altered, and DNA being damaged. We may have trouble detoxifying, causing a toxic buildup in our bodies as cells cannot purge their waste products, and we may become unable to properly assimilate nutrients, which can cause a large number of different symptoms and diseases over time.

The symptoms I experience when I am exposed to RF radiation include erratic spikes in blood pressure and resting pulse rate, pressure and tingling in the head, pressure behind the eyes with a sensation of my head feeling as if it were about to explode, burning of face and eyes, shortness of breath, hair loss, skin rashes, fatigue, confusion, forgetfulness, brain fog, fevers, nosebleeds, and headaches. These are followed by a couple of nights of insomnia, inability to stay asleep, twitching throughout my body in multiple places simultaneously, tightening of the muscles in the neck and shoulders, and foot and leg cramps. I also lose my ability to complete a thought, lose my train of thought, and often stop talking midsentence to figure out what I am trying to say. It was very scary to experience all of these sensations and symptoms before I figured out their cause. Now, it is frustrating and it is a burden to those around me, but at least I am learning to manage it all by reducing my exposure. It has drastically changed the course and quality of my life.

While there are a myriad of symptoms people experience when they are exposed to RF radiation, the most common are sleep disturbances, headaches, ringing in the ears, ear pain, confusion, eye pain, joint pain, dizziness, vertigo, palpitations, heart arrhythmias, high blood pressure, low blood pressure, tachycardia, bradycardia, skin problems, rashes, burning sensations, brain fog, memory loss, sweating, numbness, slurred speech, drowsiness, anxiety, irritability, depression, infertility, thyroid disorders, loss of appetite, distended abdomen, balance problems, blood sugar fluctuations, difficulty moving, and facial flushing.

We are electrochemical and electromagnetic beings. Our cell membranes are electrically charged. Many of our organs and systems, such as our heart, brain, muscles, intestines, and nervous system, work on natural electrical impulses. It makes sense that manmade electrical interference could ultimately disrupt these systems over time. There is also evidence to suggest that birds, bees, and vegetation are adversely affected by RFs. The rapidly declining bee population and colony collapse are getting worldwide attention because bees are responsible for pollinating the majority of the crops that then become our food.

The big question is whether we will be able to adapt to these manmade frequencies during our lifetime. I don't have the answer, but I don't suspect it will be anytime soon. This would mean that people will likely get sicker until the telecommunications industry can come up with a safer solution.

I am not a doctor or an expert on radiofrequency. I know what is true for me. I am willing to be wrong. I accept the consequences of sharing this experience and the results of my investigation. I am coming from the heart with the best of intentions to help humanity thrive. I don't believe it is safe to wait for the industries or government to take action. I intend to continue my research and publish it in an upcoming book. It is up to us to protect ourselves and our families.

## Cell Phones

The state of California issued guidelines warning people to limit their use of cell phones. It also recommends using your speakerphone and keeping the phone away from the body. This is due to the link between electromagnetic radiation and brain cancer. The World Health Organization has classified radiofrequency electromagnetic fields from mobile phones as Group 2B carcinogens, which means they are possibly carcinogenic or cause cancer in humans.

Radiofrequency is a form of electromagnetic radiation. There are two types of electromagnetic radiation. Ionizing radiation is the form of radiation emitted by X-rays, CT scans, mammograms, and radon. Ionizing radiation is known to cause cancer. There are natural and manmade sources of nonionizing radiation. Nonionizing radiation is emitted naturally as visible and ultraviolet light produced by the sun. Manmade sources come from electricity, electromagnetic fields, and microwaves. They are emitted by any appliances that have electricity running through them and by wireless devices such as cell phones and Wi-Fi routers. Scientists do not agree that nonionizing radiation in itself causes cancer.

As a former research scientist who has worked on studies that have been published in peer-reviewed scientific journals, and as a former editor for scientific papers submitted for publication to scientific journals, I can tell you that it is difficult to study the effects of radiofrequency on the body. The study must be done over the long term, over many years and even over decades. Technology changes so frequently that it is hard to design a truly meaningful study. 5G technology is about to roll out as I write this book. We have no idea what the impact will be.

It is also impossible to shield the control group. If they can find people for control groups who do not use cell phones, they have to consider that those people are constantly being bombarded with radiofrequencies from other sources, such as Wi-Fi, microwave ovens, smart meters, and other people's cell phones. If a person is a control subject in a cell phone study and does not use a cell phone but stands in front of their microwave oven as they heat their lunch, sleeps ten feet away from a smart meter, has a cordless phone in their home, or rides in a car, bus, or train where other people are using cell phones, they may develop some of the same symptoms as those subjects using those phones. That negates the impact of those symptoms in the cell phone users in the study. It is simply impossible to have a true control group to compare in these tests because there are no unexposed members of society. Therefore the results of the study are not really valid.

It is disconcerting that the cell phone industry denies most claims. Cell phone manufacturers warn that you should hold your phone no less than five-eighths of an inch away from your body, but most people do not read the fine print. If the industry issued warnings on phones, many people would use their phones the same way, just as is the case with warnings on tobacco products. There are billions of cell phone users in the world today. The truth is most people do not know there is a danger lurking around their phones and devices and would take some precautions if they did. Cell phone sales would probably remain the same even with the warnings, but at least people would know to protect themselves. Many people, especially teenagers, are on their phones constantly and even sleep with their phones on their bed, next to their bed, or even under their pillow.

One fact that most everyone can agree on is that cell phones are not meant to be touching our bodies. Holding them to your head while talking or carrying them in your pocket or your bra can cause harm by heating your tissue and subjecting you to high levels of RF radiation. It is no surprise that we are seeing a huge spike in the number of cases of brain tumors. I am aware of several people who have developed primary cancers in the thumbs of their dominant texting hand. Cell phones pose a serious threat to our health over the long term and precautions should be taken to keep them at a distance from our bodies.

We need more truly independent research that is done over long periods of time. This will take many years. Meanwhile, take precautions to protect yourself. Take this information and use common sense. We all need to be smart about the issue of radiation exposure and exercise caution whenever possible.

When I began measuring the radiofrequencies coming from these devices, I found the levels they emit are allowed levels. It is "normal" for these devices to emit such levels and is possibly necessary for them to work as they do. After becoming mindful and shielding many of my devices, I would measure levels in my home for extended periods to find out what type of spikes I would see. One day I left the house and remembered I left my radiofrequency meter running on my dining room table. When I got to my destination, I texted my son and asked him to let me know the highest level recorded since I had turned on the meter. He replied to my text that the maximum reading was 250 $\mu W/m^2$ (microwatts per meter squared). Immediately after, he sent another text saying when he sent me that text, he was near the meter and the meter reading jumped up to 1,827,000 $\mu W/m^2$, the upper limit of my meter. This spike came from his sending the text message. Just imagine if you were exposed to radiation levels thousands of times higher than the highest level in your home each time you sent or received a text message. In response to this, I switch my cell phone to airplane mode and only take it out of airplane mode a few minutes at a time if I need to use the phone or check my messages. If I need to make a call from my cell phone, I use speakerphone. If I am in a place where it is not appropriate to use the speaker, I hold my phone several inches from my face and I can still hear the other person and they can hear me. I keep all cell phone calls to a minimum length. If I am going to be on a lengthy call, I use my corded landline phone.

Prior to figuring this out, I was considering giving up my privilege to drive. I had made several very dangerous moves that could have caused me and others harm. I could not think clearly and found myself really second-guessing my driving. I found I was becoming afraid to make left turns across traffic because I didn't trust my judgment. I had this profound sense of brain fog when I drove. On one occasion I went through a red light and didn't realize I had until I got through the intersection. This sense of horror came over me as I realized what I had done. The best way I can describe the sensation in my head when a phone is on in a car is similar to when someone cracks open one car window while you are driving on a highway. There is an annoying and irritating percussion and vibration in your head. You have to open another window to make it stop. In the case where a cell phone causes this sensation, opening a window does not help. My brain feels as if it is heating up. I begin to feel nauseous.

After finding out how high the readings were coming from my cell phone, I began to question if my phone was impacting my driving. Further research gave me a clear understanding that cell phones are constantly looking for towers while you are driving and that is when they give off large spikes of radiation. I confirmed this by taking RF meter measurements while driving with cell phones on and with cell phones off. I now make certain my phone is in airplane mode whenever I am in a car. When I am driving others, I ask them to put their phones on airplane mode as well. The brain fog while I am driving is now reduced by about 90 to 95 percent.

I am concerned about autonomous cars or those enabled as Wi-Fi hotspots or synced to your phone giving off high levels of radiofrequencies. Finding a car with the lowest radiation levels will be my number-one criteria when it comes time to buy a new car.

According to the FCC, "Radiofrequency radiation, especially at microwave frequencies, can transfer energy to water molecules." This is why microwave ovens heat food and why cell phones can heat up your skin and brain tissue. This brings up the concern that there may be implications of having microwave cell towers on top of municipal water towers. This could potentially be restructuring the water molecules. This concern warrants further study by an objective source.

There have been many studies indicating that RFs pose a serious threat to our health. You have to decide how much risk you are willing to take.

## Tips to Reduce Your Radiofrequency Exposure

According to some building biologists, any levels above 10 $\mu W/m^2$ cause considerable concern. While there is no truly safe level, studies suggest you should not sleep in an area with an RF reading over 5 $\mu W/m^2$. It is critical to your health that you reduce your exposure while you sleep. While you sleep, your body is working to heal and restore itself. That said, this section should help you draw on and implement some of the most valuable tips to reduce your RF exposure and live healthier.

Within a four-mile radius of my house, there are fifty-seven cell towers and 371 RF-emitting antennas. New cell antennas are being installed on light posts, telephone poles, traffic signals, and commercial buildings as part of a distributed antenna system (DAS). It will take a long time to undo all of this infrastructure. It might take years for engineers in the industry to figure out a way to replace it with a newer, safer technology that meets the demand for innovation. Meanwhile, be smart. While it is impossible to control what goes on outside of our homes, we can control the amount of radiofrequency we generate within our homes.

If you must keep your cell phone on when you sleep, turn up the volume and keep it as far away as possible. Keep your cell phone and devices in airplane mode when you can. While your phone is in this mode, you cannot send or receive calls or text messages or use the Internet. Other phone features, such as the camera and alarms, will work while it is in airplane mode.

Ask your electric provider not to install a smart meter on your home. Some municipalities will charge to remove the meter and a monthly service fee if you opt out of a smart meter and use an analog meter instead. Be sure the analog meter that is used in its place does not emit radiofrequencies. Some analog meters have a chip in them and will still remotely send data to the carrier. If you rent your home or cannot avoid the meter, buy a shield or supplies—aluminum screening, duct tape, and a copper wire—to make your own smart meter shield. This will reduce the radiation but will not eliminate it. The meter will still transmit your information to a microwave tower and to your utility company.

If you live near a cell tower, take extra precautions. I've taken consistently high readings in people's homes that were several hundred feet away from the tower. Readings are consistently in the range of 300 to 500 $\mu W/m^2$ with all phones and Wi-Fi turned off. A 2002 study suggests RF-related symptoms are highest within 200 yards of a cell tower.

For comparison, the background level in my home is about 2 $\mu W/m^2$ with everything that produces radiofrequency turned off. Even with my smart meter shielded, I get random spikes that I assume are from either my smart meter or my neighbors' smart meters in the range of 1,000 to 44,000 $\mu W/m^2$. A smart meter can transmit data thousands of times per day, causing random spikes at harmful levels.

When I had the cordless digital phones and base charging station in my home, my background readings were in the range of 300 $\mu W/m^2$ throughout the house. The levels near the base were extremely high.

Even if you are not experiencing any symptoms from your exposure to radiofrequencies, your body is still impacted. Technology will only continue to expand, and as our devices and appliances become "smarter" and faster, our exposure will increase. Over time I believe everyone will develop symptoms to varying degrees. The time to take precautions is not after you have advanced disease processes in your body. The time to act is now.

Most people don't have the time to do their own research. There have been many studies done on RFs. It is often difficult to understand all the scientific jargon and to weed out the industry bias. Here are some precautionary actions you can take to reduce your RF exposure and protect yourself and your family:

- *Get rid of any cordless landline digital phones in your house. These cause very high levels of RFs and are one of the easiest changes to make. Replace them with corded phones.*
- *Keep your cell phone and wireless devices on airplane mode as often as possible.*
- *All phones in your car should be on airplane mode unless you need one for navigating. Consider using physical maps or printing directions at home prior to getting in the car.*
- *Keep your cell phone and devices away from your body. Set your phone on a surface and use a stylus.*
- *Use speakerphone when possible.*
- *Limit the number and length of calls from your cell phones and Bluetooth devices.*

- *Do not sleep with any cordless or Wi-Fi enabled devices in your bedroom or sleeping area.*
- *Do not use fitness monitoring bracelets.*
- *Keep all of these devices as far away from you as possible when you are not using them.*
- *Do not hold laptops on your lap. Use them on a desk or table.*
- *Keep cell phones and tablets from young children. Radiofrequencies are more dangerous to their developing bodies and brains.*
- *If you must use a wireless baby monitor, keep it as far as possible from your baby's crib or children's beds.*
- *Read real books in place of electronic books. If you must use an electronic reader, use airplane mode.*
- *Opt out of having a smart meter on your home or use a smart meter shield.*
- *Do not use smart thermostats.*
- *Opt for analog home appliances over smart appliances. Smart appliances send signals that communicate with your smart meter.*
- *Turn off the Wi-Fi on your computer whenever possible. Use ethernet cables to connect to your router or minimize the time you are connected to your wireless network.*
- *Turn off your Wi-Fi router when you are sleeping. If you need to keep it on to keep your phones or alarm system working, keep the router and devices as far from you as possible.*

- *Consider shielding the devices that emit EMFs or RF radiation. You may need to hire a professional to help.*
- *Do not live near a cell tower. If you must, adequately shield your home.*

Each of these is one small step in the right direction to reduce your exposure to the many varieties of RF. As you implement these small changes, you'll notice changes across the board. The good news is that I have shared this information with a number of people who have taken some of these preventive measures to reduce exposure. I have received great feedback from them. In some cases, their health issues or mystery symptoms have resolved or improved.

## Tips to Reduce Body Voltage and EMF Exposure

Both EMF and RF radiation stress the body, cause biological effects, and raise body voltage. To understand what sort of things increase body voltage most, I took measurements all around my house and other people's houses measuring multiple voltages. I also loaned my meters to several others who took measurements in their homes and workplaces. Body voltage is consistently higher when the person is in areas of high EMF or RF radiation. Taking just a couple of steps away from those areas will significantly reduce body voltage. It is important to note that distance is your friend. The best thing you can do is distance yourself from those things that raise your voltage, even if it is just by a few extra inches.

To illustrate, when I am working on my laptop, my body voltage decreases simply by taking the following actions: I move the laptop about six inches farther away from me on the table and ensure the cord is not near my feet or legs. I often use the laptop on battery power only. I also turn my Wi-Fi off on my computer when I don't need to use the Internet. If I am on a website or listening to a webinar replay, I have found that I can turn off the Wi-Fi and continue to read or listen as long as I don't change pages while I am disconnected from my wireless network. I take my hands off the laptop whenever I am reading from the computer. I will often zoom to make the text a little larger and move the laptop even farther away. I have also purchased a USB keyboard so that I can type with the laptop farther away. It was a ten-dollar investment that has made a big difference. When possible I use an Ethernet cable to connect my computer directly to my modem so I can use the Internet without Wi-Fi.

It may seem like a lot of effort, but it is simply a matter of being mindful. Taking a few small steps may reduce your risk significantly. Think about the placement of your electronics in your home. If you use an alarm clock, where is it? Is it inches away from your head? Can you move it to the far side of the nightstand or perhaps across the room? If it is near your bed, where does the cord run? If it runs behind your bed to an outlet near your head, is there another outlet you can plug into that is farther from your bed? If you must have items plugged in at close proximity to your bed, unplug them before you go to sleep. Some people even install switches to turn off the breakers or simply switch off the breakers supplying all power to their bedrooms at night. Just be sure your refrigerator, furnace, submersible pumps, or other critical electronics are not on the same circuit breaker.

Be aware of what is on the other side of the wall where you spend the most time. EMFs and RFs pass through walls and floors. Rearrange furniture in your home and workspace so you are at a safer distance from things such as breaker boxes, fuse panels, refrigerators, air conditioning units, and other devices or industrial equipment that may give off large amounts of stray electricity.

Here are some additional steps you can take to reduce your body voltage and EMF exposure:

- *Take the precautionary actions to reduce RF exposure as stated above.*
- *Avoid fluorescent light fixtures. If you have them in your home, I suggest investing to replace them. If they are in your workspace and you have natural light, can you turn the lights off and have enough light to work or add a desk lamp? In some cases, the lights are on multiple banks and you can turn half of them off.*
- *Avoid compact fluorescent lamp (CFL) lights. In addition to putting off high levels of EMFs and high-frequency radiation that is absorbed by your body, they contain*

*mercury, which causes a serious threat to the environment that far outweighs the benefit of being energy efficient.*

- *Avoid LED lightbulbs. They contain lead, arsenic, and heavy metals. They also emit high levels of EMFs. Use incandescent bulbs when possible. Full-spectrum lightbulbs are good alternatives but are more expensive.*
- *Replace dimmer switches with standard light switches.*
- *Organize power cords so they are not near your body. Run power cords behind your desk instead of near your feet.*
- *Unplug electronic devices when not in use. This also reduces your electrical consumption, your electric bill, and reduces your carbon footprint.*
- *Consider putting filters on your house, which reduce high frequency spikes on the electrical wiring in your home.*

RFs and EMFs pose serious threats to our well-being. Chronic exposure and increasing levels will catch up with us over time. It will serve you to implement these tips to reduce exposure.

I have no plans of going off grid if I can effectively manage my exposure. I will continue to use my devices in a much smarter and more cognizant manner. As I reduced my use of my cell phone and Internet, my symptoms have begun to resolve. Not only have I noticed an increase in my health and well-being, but I feel more in the moment and am experiencing life at a higher level.

I realized I was spending a lot more time on my devices and social media than I needed to in order to maintain my connections and interactions with others. It was passing time, but it was not contributing to my life in any meaningful way. I now have a lot more free time to live life and enjoy others in person. For that reason alone, it is worth disconnecting more regularly. Consider that the time we spend connected to technology is time we are disconnected from the present moment and from those we are with, including our children, family, and friends.

## Lessons from a Radio-Free Retreat

I decided to finish writing this book in a remote area of West Virginia with no cell towers and strict regulations on radiofrequency devices. I spent a week as disconnected as I could while maintaining a somewhat normal lifestyle. I had minimal exposures to RFs that were outside of my control. These included intermittent exposure to Wi-Fi when I went to town, cars passing by with Smart technology, and cell phones. Even though there are no cell towers there, if a phone or device is left on, it is consistently sending out RF signals searching for a tower.

I noticed significant improvements in my health over the course of the week. My energy level increased, and my vision improved. The twitching throughout my body and the leg cramps stopped completely. I found it easy to carry on conversations, I had clearer thoughts, and I could effectively verbalize my words. I did not experience any of the tingling or burning in my head or pressure behind my eyes that had been pretty constant for months. My average resting pulse rate decreased from 125 beats per minute to seventy-four beats per minute. My average blood pressure decreased from 130/81 to 112/68. I truly felt like myself again.

I had the privilege of meeting and interviewing other electrosensitive people from around the country who came to this area to seek refuge from RFs. Their stories were eerily similar to mine. Many claim their symptoms began upon the installation of their smart meters. I am not concluding that smart meters are responsible for all of these problems. Perhaps the strong pulses they emit put our overburdened bodies over the edge.

Each source of radiation has unique frequencies and different pulsations. Not everyone experiences the same symptoms or reacts similarly. Some react only to specific frequencies. Some react only to certain devices and appliances. Some can have Wi-Fi but cannot tolerate cell phones. Some can tolerate specific cell phone carriers but not others. Some cannot tolerate any radiofrequency whatsoever. Regardless of the type of sensitivities each of these people experience, they are finding the solutions they need to restore their health and peace of mind.

I struggle with the realization that this radiation will cause suffering for many people and animals. The fact that everyone has different reactions to different exposures makes it nearly impossible to evaluate. Conventional science will have a hard time studying this and getting repeatable results. Medical schools may not train doctors to identify this problem. It is not likely that we will see independent studies with true control groups. Sadly, most of this technology has been rolled out without ever having been studied for safety to our health. Many of the people who are being harmed will not find the cause unless we can share this information far and wide.

The health benefits I gained from that retreat lasted several weeks. The symptoms then returned in full force. I am managing my life responsibilities by strategically taking radio-free retreats so I can function when I need to. For now, I have found I need a few days completely disconnected from all technology about once per month. I have found a cabin in the woods closer to my home where I am protected from radiofrequency radiation. I am experimenting with homeopathic remedies and finding the balance that best supports me. I will continue to share as I learn.

## Putting This in Context

Until I can make a blanket statement about what we have to do to overcome this, we must remember that we are here to live our unique journeys. We have tremendous power to influence how we experience our lives and our health.

We are complex beings. In addition to our physical bodies, we are electromagnetic fields. We have incredible power to co-create our physical existence. I believe my experience with EHS occurred to teach me to take better care of myself amidst this technology so I can help others as this becomes a problem for more and more of us. I feel I am at the forefront of contributing to the solution.

If you are experiencing symptoms, understand that there are many methods and modalities that can help you. There is not a one-size-fits-all solution. The most important thing you can do is minimize your exposure and eliminate those sources to which you react. This may require you to do some experimenting and journaling of your symptoms. You must then focus your efforts on self-care and supporting the needs of your mind and body.

As society moves to a place of acceptance and begins to realize the impact this manmade radiation is having on our bodies, it is important to understand several things. For those who are electrosensitive or experience EHS, you may find people don't believe you, your doctors may not validate your concerns, you may be labeled as "crazy," your relationships may suffer, your marriage may be tested, and you may find yourself feeling afraid and isolated. For those who have someone in your life who has EHS, realize their condition is fragile. This is real. Respect their need to be protected. Turn off your devices when you are around them, and support them the best you can. Every text message you send or receive contributes to this electromagnetic pollution. Every cellular call you make irradiates everyone around you. Use your devices ethically. Knowledge is crucial. There are ways to manage this. Together, we will find solutions.

# Chapter 6

## Ethical Consumerism and Environmental Responsibility

When I was about twelve, I became interested in photography. I used to go on nature walks and take pictures. One day while taking pictures at a nature preserve, I saw a sign coming up out of the ground that was fashioned to look like a tombstone. The title read *Obituary: Earth, Birthplace of Mankind*. The words on that tombstone went on to outline all of the ways man destroyed Earth through carelessness and lack of concern for its well-being. As I stood in front of that sign, tears streamed down my face. In that moment, I decided I would do all I could to be part of the solution, not the problem. I wasn't sure what I could do, or even how I could do it. However, I knew I couldn't stand by and watch our beautiful home meet its demise. It felt as if I was being called to contribute to the healing of the planet while becoming a steward for the environment. I became increasingly interested in nature, sustainability, and the environment. That started a journey for me, and I eventually became an activist and obtained a degree in environmental biology. Now, more than ever, my journey continues as I work to become an active and valuable part of the solution.

Ethical consumerism and environmental responsibility starts with each of us. It might not take a dramatic obituary for the Earth to change your behaviors, but the small steps we each take can add up to make a remarkable difference in the overall health of our society, starting with the Earth.

It may feel easier to be comfortably unaware than to take a stand. We can no longer turn the other cheek and leave it up to someone else to protect or save our planet. We are destroying our Earth and the essence of that which supports us. Simply by being a part of the population, we are contributing to the problem. To thrive in this century, we must revert to respecting nature and establish a sense of connection to the Earth. We are evolving individually and collectively, whether we realize it or not. We have no choice but to reduce our footprint. There is no time to wait for others to do it. We cannot depend on regulatory agencies to mandate it. We can't solve these problems individually, but collectively we can take small, consistent steps in the right direction. We can all make those shifts that lead to substantial change.

Nature is quite resilient and can generally repair itself, but only if we stop causing the harm. Collectively, we can change these trends when we implement conservation efforts and are good stewards of the environment. We often don't realize the impact of our choices. Each choice we make with respect to water, clothing, what we put in and on our bodies, the environment we live in, and what we spend our money on has consequences to our health and the environment. As you become more educated, you can make better choices and treat your body and the Earth with a higher level of respect. Once we know the implications of purchasing certain types of food or products, we have the responsibility to make ethical choices. When we purchase something that is produced in a way that is not in integrity with our values, we are consciously deciding to support those industries and practices.

This chapter will help you identify your imprint on the world and find ways to reduce the damage you may unintentionally cause.

## Recycling and Reducing Waste

As a society, we are generating more waste than our Earth can handle. We are transporting garbage extraordinarily long distances and even across state lines. This is caused by a lack of space in large cities, so we have to literally outsource our garbage dumping. This has to change. Together, it is time to work to reduce the amount of garbage we generate. Recycle anything you can, but even more critically, avoid using disposable items whenever possible. It takes a village, and each piece of trash we do not create is one less piece of trash for which we have to account.

Of all the garbage we generate, plastic pollution is of particular concern. In the United States alone, we use nearly fifty billion plastic water bottles each year. The majority of water bottles are not even recycled. A water bottle can take hundreds of years to decompose, so they are literally piling up on top of one another. That plastic is then causing harm to the environment and wildlife. Whenever possible, use an alternative like a drinking container made of glass or stainless steel. Be sure to periodically wash out your water bottles, and let them dry completely between uses to reduce fungal and bacterial contamination. Reusing and recycling are just a start.

Even when we can put our waste into a recycling program, it is not always recycled and is not fully reused. If you throw nonrecyclable garbage or food in with your recyclables, they generally will not be recycled. When you put things that are not recyclable in the recycling bin, in many cases the entire lot is kicked out and will not be recycled. The best way to avoid this is to educate yourself on the local practices of your recycling and garbage disposal company. For instance, if you recycle your mail and keep the cellophane windows on your envelopes, all of your paper waste may not get recycled. If you replace the metal lid on a glass jar before putting it in your recycle bin, chances are the whole jar will not get recycled. In fact, the entire bin or bag may go to the landfill instead of being recycled. It just takes a little effort to get it right, and a little can go a long way.

In many cases, it is acceptable to leave labels on glass jars or bottles, but labels must be removed from plastic or tin cans before they can be recycled. Knowledge is key to ensure you are practicing sound recycling. When possible, repurpose nondisposable items or find them another home. If you no longer have use for them, consider selling or donating the items. We all have a responsibility to make a difference in the waste we create. Be conscientious, thoughtful, and invest that little bit of extra energy to ensure you get it right.

## Water

We have a fixed amount of water on Earth. It may change form, but we cannot increase what we have at any point in time. It may exist in liquid form in our bodies and our waterways, in the form of humidity, condensation, or vapor in our atmosphere, or frozen in the form of snow or in our ice caps. Tragically, the toxins that accumulate over time are increasingly contaminating our water. The longer it takes us to realize we are poisoning our life source, the more difficult it will be to correct the damage.

While I was in college in the 1980s and while interning in a toxicology lab with the US Fish and Wildlife Service, we conducted a lot of water quality analyses. At that time there were numerous estrogens and estrogen-mimicking materials in the water, largely from the use of birth control pills and agricultural runoff from livestock treated with hormones. Because of this, experts predicted that within a few decades we would not have fish in our waters since those fish were becoming androgynous and unable to reproduce because of the havoc caused by the hormones in the water. It is possible these hormones in our diet and in our water are disrupting our endocrine systems and are contributing to the sharp rise in the level of breast cancer in both men and women, early onset puberty, infertility, and imbalances of hormones in our bodies.

Water treatment facilities generally filter out solid waste and then treat the water for pathogens such as bacteria and viruses and to protect us from waterborne disease. These facilities often use chlorine or other disinfectants to accomplish this. Municipal water supplies are stringently tested, but most people don't realize that the acceptable limits are constantly changing to make the water fit to drink. For instance, when levels of chlorine in the water are not killing all the parasites and bacteria, more chlorine is added and the acceptable range of chlorine is continually raised so that it meets standards. Our water is not meeting the same standards it did several years ago. It is now a moving target, and we are seeing an increase in higher levels of potentially dangerous chemicals in the water. These compounds kill our normal gut flora, which are the good bacteria that aid our digestive and immune systems.

I was shocked to learn that chemicals and drugs are not filtered out of our municipal water supply. They build up over time. There are acceptable levels of each toxic chemical such as pesticides, lead, fluoride, and drugs. The acceptable levels of many of them keep going up to ensure our water meets the standards.

Over five billion pounds of pesticides are used worldwide each year. These chemicals either run off into the groundwater, accumulate in the environment, or are taken up by the crops via absorption or via their root system. We then eat the pesticides in the produce, some of the pesticides accumulate in our bodies, and some are filtered out and excreted from our bodies. You cannot be assured that any chemical with which you make contact is safe. All chemicals are considered safe until proven otherwise. If a chemical is not acutely toxic, it may be considered safe. Sadly, it is too costly to conduct the studies to prove toxicity. In most cases, testing is left up to the companies that are manufacturing and selling the chemical. There is no incentive, and the company could lose profit if the chemical proved to be toxic. As a result, many chemicals go untested.

Interactions occur between all the chemicals in our water, the metals in our plumbing that leach into the water, and the materials that are used to solder the pipes. Many interactions occur from the time the water is tested at a source to the time it gets to the faucet in your home. Even if your home is on a well, contaminants in the ground water and potential risks of interactions with your plumbing materials exist.

The chemicals we put down our drains eventually end up in our drinking water. While we can't control what others do, we can reduce our footprint with our choices. Many toxic chemicals in clothing do not get filtered out in the municipal water treatment facilities. Many people get sick from shopping in stores because of the off-gassing of chemicals on the fabric. When we wash laundry, many of these toxic materials, such as formaldehyde, go down the drain into our water supply.

Plastic microbeads from personal care products—and plastic fibers that are shed from microfiber fabrics that go down our drains—are of particular concern. Fibers break off microfiber fabrics while they are being laundered. The more frequently you wash these fabrics and the longer their wash and dry cycle, the more fibers you contribute to the environment. These small beads and fibers pass through water filtration systems and enter the environment, where they are ingested by fish and shellfish. They cause harm to these species, accumulate in the food chain, and eventually end up in our food supply. Avoiding the use of synthetic fabrics and microfibers, reducing the amount you wash them, and avoiding products with microbeads is a good start.

These are some compounds that end up in our water supply:

- *Medications and drugs that you ingest that pass through your system and are excreted in your urine, as well as those ingested by the rest of the population*
- *Runoff of agricultural pesticides that get into the groundwater*
- *Hormones, pesticides, and antibiotics that pass through livestock*

- *Materials that you apply to your skin, which are absorbed and enter your bloodstream*
- *Detergents, bleach, and fabric softeners that you use in washing your laundry*
- *Plastic fibers that break off of microfiber and synthetic fabrics while laundering*
- *The chemicals on your clothing, toxic dyes, fire retardants, water repellents, antimicrobial chemicals, pesticides, and preservatives that are discharged into the wastewater*
- *Anything you put in the drain, including cleaning products and antibacterial soaps*
- *Chemicals you use on your lawn including pesticides and fertilizers*

When we leave the safety of our drinking water to a government agency, we can be assured that we will not become acutely ill from a pathogen, but there are no guarantees regarding the long-term impact of ingesting all of these chemicals. Are you comfortable ingesting even small amounts of poison in every glass of water you drink?

I do not believe there is any source of pristine water left on the planet. I recommend everyone filter his or her tap water. It is important to filter out toxic chemicals from the water you ingest as well as the water you bathe in. At a minimum, a pitcher type filter is inexpensive and reduces chlorine and lead from the water you drink. Request a copy of your local water supplier's water quality report to find out which chemicals and disinfection products are in your water at the source. If your municipality uses monochloramine to disinfect your water, you need to research each specific filter because many remove chlorine but not monochloramine. I prefer reverse osmosis, because it removes any chemicals, fluoride, and all particles from the water. Removing particles also eliminates radiation contamination. Reverse osmosis also removes minerals so it is important that you consume a good balance of minerals in your diet.

Many levels of filtration are available, and it depends on your location, your water source, and your budget. I have municipal water that is heavily chlorinated and fluoridated, and have galvanized pipes in my structure that was built about 1970. I have a whole-house chlorine and solids filter, which costs about forty dollars, charcoal/KDF filters to remove chlorine on each showerhead, which cost about forty dollars each, and a good three-step reverse osmosis system in my kitchen that costs about $150 plus the cost of installation. Each of these requires filter changes about every six months, but steadily increases the water quality in my home.

## Treatment of Animals and Agricultural Concerns

Environmental organizations and regulatory agencies are failing our ecosystems and each of us. They are often turning the other cheek as politics play a bigger role in some of the organizations. Then, big business is spending huge amounts of money to cover up the truth. The fact that the truth is being hidden does not change the outcome. It is critically important that we educate ourselves and do all we can to keep a healthy environment and food supply.

Our food supply is in serious danger. Pesticides are contaminating our crops. Some of our food sources have been genetically modified to the extent that our bodies no longer recognize them as food. Livestock is raised in horrific conditions. Many fish populations are in danger of extinction due to overexploitation and contamination with pesticides and hormones. Bees are becoming endangered and most crops depend on them for pollination.

Agricultural chemicals and pesticides have penetrated our water and our food supply. Washing produce doesn't remove all of the chemicals. The chemicals get into the plants via absorption and are taken up by the roots.

Animals are often raised in inhumane, overcrowded conditions. Some animals will never see daylight in their lifetime, living knee-deep in their own feces. Others, like chickens, are confined to small cages or crates that are stacked on top of one another. It is not only cruel to the animal, but the food probably does not contain a lot of vital nutrients after being raised under these conditions. These confined animal-feeding operations are also contributing to the problem of antibiotic-resistant bacteria.

Dairy cows are often injected with hormones so they produce much more milk than they were ever intended to produce naturally. The mechanical action of the milking machines causes the cow's teats to become raw, bleed, and become infected. They require constant antibiotics to fight the infection from living in these conditions. The majority of antibiotics used in the United States are administered to livestock and farm animals that we end up ingesting. Both synthetic and naturally occurring hormones are present in animal's meat and waste. The hormones and antibiotics pass through to the milk and some is excreted in their urine. This urine eventually ends up back in the water cycle.

The truth is we probably can't sustainably raise enough organic, grass-fed dairy, grass-fed beef, and free-range poultry to feed the population of the planet. We must reduce the amount of animal products we consume to prevent the horrific conditions required to meet the massive demand.

Agricultural animals contribute significantly to methane emissions and global warming. We must reduce our consumption of animal products. If your diet is high in animal products, consider going meat and dairy free one day per week. Reduce your portion sizes of meat and increase your produce intake. Start small. Choose poultry or other sources of protein over beef. Replace milk with almond or coconut milk. Then work to further reduce your consumption of dairy and meat products, and only enjoy those products from locally sourced or organic farms.

You get adequate amounts of protein in your diet without consuming animal products. Many people reverse health conditions simply by eliminating meat and dairy products from their diet. You may be surprised to see how much better you feel if you remove animal products from your diet for a week or two.

**Your Personal Products and Environment**

Your body and your home are your sanctuary. Use care to make choices that support a healthy body, lifestyle, and home. Be conscientious about the products you put on your body. Anything you apply to yourself, such as lotion, makeup, perfumes or colognes, soaps, and chemicals in your water can be absorbed through your skin.

Products applied to the skin can be more toxic than if we were to ingest them. If you were to ingest any of these products, your liver would work to detoxify the product. When a product or water is absorbed into your skin, it enters your bloodstream without detoxification. Your kidneys will then have to filter it from your blood, but there is a much higher level of toxicity and impact to your body. The FDA does not require personal products to post all ingredients, so do your best to use products with the least amount of chemicals in them. If you wouldn't ingest them, then don't put them on your body. For instance, you can use coconut or almond oil with an optional drop of an organic essential oil in place of commercial body lotion; you can brush your teeth with coconut oil instead of toothpastes that contain dyes, artificial sweeteners, and fluoride; and you can clean most surfaces in your home with vinegar.

Many chemicals and personal care products such as lotion and soap are tested on animals. As a scientist, I conducted studies to determine efficacy and lethal dosages and lethal concentrations of anesthetics on fish. Other than a few that I rescued for my personal aquarium, I can tell you that I put thousands of fish to death. Even those that survived the experiments, including the control animals, were put to death after the study. There are ethical concerns with respect to this inhumane practice of animal testing. In most cases, a lethal concentration of the product ingredients needs to be determined and high doses are administered to test animals to determine which levels are actually toxic. Animals needlessly suffer and are often put to death at the end of the testing. Buy from companies that do not test their products on animals.

But it doesn't stop there. Consider not only what you eat and the products you use but also the environment in which you reside. Take steps to make your personal environment safer and more energetically peaceful. Consider feng shui, a practice in which you observe your surroundings and shift the energy simply by placing your possessions in a manner that brings harmony to your home and your life.

Taking even the simplest steps, like removing your shoes when you enter your home, can have a substantial impact on your environment. Think about it for a second. Everything you step on ends up on the bottom of your shoes. I once worked in a research center where radiation studies were done. I did not work in a radiation lab or with radioactive chemicals. On occasion we would take a Geiger counter and measure levels of radioactivity around the building. Much to my surprise, my shoes set off the detector on two occasions. The only way I could have picked up the radiation on my shoes was from walking in the same hallways as other scientists who worked in the radiation labs. While most of you probably don't work around radiation, think about where your shoes have been. Think about how often we might step on bird poop, bug guts, worms, and fallout from aerial sources, pollution, pollen, chemicals, or germs. You do not want to be tracking these things into your home, especially if you have children or pets.

In review, there are many small steps you can take that will create substantial changes. It doesn't take drastic transformation to improve your well-being and that of the planet. Pick a few goals and then implement them. Share them with your friends and notice how even the smallest of shifts can make substantial changes.

## Contributing to the Solution

Margaret Mead once said, "Never doubt that a small group of thoughtful, committed citizens can change the world.

Indeed, it is the only thing that ever has." When concerned citizens decide to boycott certain types of food or services, we influence the market and have the power to change industries and practices globally. As consumers, we carry tremendous power to shift market practices and attitudes. We don't have time to wait for politicians to agree on the issues. The fate of our world is in our hands. Here are ways you can reduce the impact of your actions on the world:

- *Buy products that are not tested on animals.*
- *Eliminate or reduce the amount of milk and dairy products you consume.*
- *Reduce the amount of animal products you consume.*
- *Buy organic.*
- *Use any animal products that you buy, and do not let them expire or go to waste.*
- *Use products on your skin that are safe enough to eat.*
- *Stop buying disposable water bottles. Refill and reuse bottles.*
- *Use reusable grocery bags or corrugated bins in place of disposable plastic shopping bags.*
- *Know the requirements for recycling, and follow them strictly or don't bother recycling.*
- *Repurpose, sell, or donate items you no longer need.*
- *Do not put expired over-the-counter or prescription medications in the garbage or flush them down the toilet. Dispose of them properly.*
- *Replace antibacterial soap with regular soap.*

- *Know which food is genetically engineered and buy non-GMO food.*
- *Buy cage-free, free-range, or organic poultry products.*
- *Buy grass-fed or organic meat when possible.*
- *Grow your own fruit, vegetables, and herbs if you can.*
- *Use nontoxic laundry products, free of harsh chemicals, dyes, and perfumes.*
- *Avoid buying synthetic fabrics that are made from microfibers.*
- *Opt for natural fiber clothing when possible.*
- *Filter your drinking water, and fill your bottles from your own source.*
- *Use sustainable products whenever possible.*
- *Use nontoxic cleaning products such as vinegar and baking soda.*
- *If you use diapers, use cloth diapers when possible.*
- *If you use disposable diapers, dump any solid waste into the toilet before putting the diaper in the garbage.*
- *Combine errands to reduce the amount of miles you drive.*
- *Rainforests, coral reefs, and the oceans act as a buffer to damage that is done to the environment. Whenever possible, support organizations that protect these fragile ecosystems.*

Remember that by purchasing food or products, we support the practices that are being used to produce them and keep them on the supermarket shelves. Rome wasn't built in a day. It takes a lot of time and collective energy to reverse the damage we have caused through years of action, but it can be done. Choose two to three implementables from this list, and make them part of your everyday life. You then become part of the solution, and you are supporting the same universe that supports you.

# Section II

# Mindset, Miracles, and the Spiritual Nature of Healing

We are hungry for change but often fear taking steps to create lasting impact. Some of us are not willing to go through the discomfort of stepping out of our comfort zone. We want to heal but don't always have the necessary components to do so. We want the world to be a better place but feel our contribution will be too insignificant or we don't want to take responsibility and action.

Mindset, emotional state, and spirituality are often overlooked in healing. Through my experiences, I have learned a tremendous amount about how we can enhance our capacity to heal at a fundamental level. I have come to believe that we have more power over our health than we realize.

In this section we will explore the missing components of healing, the power of belief and intention, and the importance of implementing self-care and spiritual practices into our lives.

# Chapter 7

# The Missing Components of Healing

I have witnessed a lot of emotional and physical healing throughout my life. In this chapter I will share why I believe people are capable of healing. Even though I did not know what I did at the time, I was able to reverse engineer and explain what I believe happened with my own healing over twenty-five years and from working with clients over eighteen years. Through my own experiences, I have found these components have played a big part in healing for many people.

I will discuss the importance of forgiveness, gratitude, and releasing negative emotions and influences from our lives. Shifting your vibration can change your life simply by intending to do so. I will explore the mystical nature of healing, miracles, and how shifting our mindset, opening our heart, and trusting our gut feelings can produce miracles in our lives. As we walk toward healing as a society, we will begin to realize the importance of these missing components.

## Let Go of Negative Emotions

It is widely accepted that stress is one of the leading causes of disease. East Asian cultures understand that disease comes from energetic disruptions in the body. These can come in the form of physiological or emotional disruptions. Disease can manifest from emotions such as fear, sadness, anger, apathy, and discontentment.

Emotions cause issues in the tissues. Our negative emotions, judgments, and beliefs often get in the way of our healing. Our fears stop us dead in our tracks. While our fears protect us from moving forward and keep us safe and comfortable, we need to be moving forward if we want to heal in a time of health crisis. Fear might prevent us from doing so. When we keep doing the same things to our bodies, we cannot expect the result to be different.

The majority of our thoughts are not essential. We create excessive stress with these nonessential thoughts. Obsessive thinking or worrying does not serve us. Just as we cannot fully understand the body by studying cadavers, we will never understand the mind by studying the brain.

You have much greater influence and control over your circumstances than you might initially believe. It is not only about responding to all the things you have going on around you, but doing so while being present in the moment. You might quickly feel overwhelmed if you try to control the circumstances around you and just focus on your fear of what might happen in the future.

Be okay with where you are. It will be difficult if you attach self-worth to an outcome that is outside your control. I invite you to get creative with where you are at this time in your life. Be open to seeing another way.

God or a greater power is not only outside of us, but also within. Our healing ability is limited only by our minds. Our bodies operate at a level of perfection that we may never fully grasp. We each have our own definition of perfection. It is not something we strive for that is unattainable. It is our current state.

The truth is we are all perfect in our current state. Every experience in our lives has been perfect for our growth and expansion. That perfection is sometimes disguised as drama, trauma, struggle, hardship, busy schedules, and stress. Be comfortable with who you are. Accept yourself right now as you are. Know that you have done the best you know how. An emotional scar from the past might be causing the illness you are experiencing. I have seen many cases where I've worked with clients on an emotional issue only to have their physical symptoms disappear. I have had clients ask, "Do you think I could have been creating this?" and "Could this have been causing my problem all along?" I don't have all the answers, but I believe emotional scars cause a lot more illness than we realize.

Understand that there are things within you that when left unresolved manifest as problems in your health and in relationships with others. Spend some time noticing what bothers you about other people, then reflect on ways this can be an issue for you. It may be that you have exhibited this same behavior toward someone else in the past. Perhaps it is a pattern that you repeat, or it may be that others have treated you this same way. Look at how this has made you feel, and think about other experiences this reminds you of. There is often something within you that needs to be healed. Everything we judge is a projection of something within ourselves.

When we project an issue on someone else and are blaming them, we keep perpetuating the problem. We actually give them control. When we complain about something, we are creating more of it. We create separation when we compare ourselves to someone else. Healing involves taking back your power.

Look at and learn from your emotional wounds so you can move to the next phase of your life. Allow yourself to be transformed by the challenges you have faced. Our wounds are not as much about what happened as they are about who we have become in spite of them.

Think about how you tell the stories of your life. If you are telling them from a victim perspective, you will likely reinforce that experience, stay in victim mode, and continue to blame the one you perceive to be at fault. If you tell those same stories from the perspective of what you have learned or who you have become from having lived through those experiences, you will have evolved and help others as well.

It is really all about our journey of becoming whole again. It is about releasing what no longer serves us so we can heal and allow our soul's journey to unfold. It is important that you recognize and release any destructive emotions and patterns. It is not as difficult as it sounds. Sometimes simply acknowledging the problem diminishes its power.

In her book *You Can Heal Your Life*, the late Louise Hay wrote that our thoughts create our problems and they can correct them. We are not the victims of our health problems, but the creators of them. Many of our thoughts are negative. It is when we take complete responsibility for our emotional baggage that we can be at peace and transform our health.

## The Importance of Forgiveness

We tend to hold resentment, anger, and hurt indefinitely and at a deep energetic level. Unless we have actively worked on addressing them, chances are we hold many deep-buried wounds that have never been released. This can cause disruptions in the body and can interfere with healing. We need to forgive in order to heal.

We all want to do our best. We have all hurt others in some way, whether it was a condescending remark, a laugh at someone's actions, a rolling of the eyeballs, or as a result of being painfully honest with someone. However obvious or subtle, whether it was meant to intimidate or not, we have all done it at some point. Whether intentional or not, we might have been hurt by others in the same way. We should work to forgive ourselves and others in order to come to a place of peace. Think about the Lord's Prayer that says, "Forgive us our trespasses as we forgive those who trespass against us." It is a two-way street.

Forgiving someone else is a powerful form of self-care. It is important to forgive others for any betrayal, pain, or suffering they may have caused you. If you find it impossible to forgive another person for their role in the problem, try to realize the power that forgiveness will give you. You will benefit no matter how difficult it may seem right now. When you are ready consciously or energetically, true forgiveness will come. Holding on to grudges only harms you. You continue to punish yourself when you don't forgive others.

Sometimes we feel that others do not deserve to be forgiven. If we forgive them, we believe we are letting them off the hook for the wrongs they have done. We are saying that what they did was acceptable to us. We can't control what others do or have done. The person who wronged you had some experiences that injured them. They did not grow up hoping to be hurtful, disrespectful, or manipulative. We can't control how we responded in the past or that we allowed them to hurt us. It is not up to us to judge them for their actions. We do not need to become best friends with this person or welcome them back into our lives. Everyone is at a different place in his or her evolution. The only thing we can control is when to let it go.

We can't change the past. When someone betrays you or lets you down, that anger, sadness, or resentment takes away your inner peace. If we do not forgive, we stay stuck in negative emotional patterns. It is difficult to move on when we are holding on to blame, judgment, resentment, or even hatred.

Forgive others for their judgments or advice. They often mean well, want to help you, and are operating from their beliefs and programming. It doesn't have to be in alignment with yours. Trust your gut feelings on what is best for you.

Realize that they did the best they could with what they had or what they understood at the time. Let them off the hook for what you perceive as their wrongdoings. It is important to also let yourself off the hook because you did the best you could and did what you thought was best even though you may know differently now. We all have our strengths and weaknesses. It is difficult on us and on others when we force them to live up to our expectations.

Forgive yourself for whatever you may have felt or done. When you do, you can take responsibility for it, make peace, and move on. If you don't forgive yourself, you can't move forward. You will remain stuck in the past, creating patterns that hold you there. We can't change the past. We have all made mistakes, behaved irresponsibly, hurt other's feelings, or let ourselves or others down. We have made choices that we are not satisfied with and feel we must punish ourselves. If others have hurt you, you must not only forgive them but you must forgive yourself for allowing them to hurt you. There is great power in forgiving yourself. As you forgive yourself, it will become easier to forgive others.

Forgive yourself for not taking action and for wishing you had done something differently. Take what you have learned and use it to do better moving forward. Forgive yourself for any of the choices you have made and for any role they have played in your illness. Forgive the treatment plans you chose. Forgive the medicine you took that may have caused harm. Forgive the food you have eaten that caused you distress. Forgive the companies that betrayed you.

We often hold a lifetime of trauma patterns within our bodies. This is unhealthy and impacts our physical and emotional well-being. You will not heal from emotional wounds until you forgive yourself and anyone else you feel has contributed to or caused those wounds. This step frees us emotionally and clears energetic blockages that keep us from healing physically. Sometimes, we move away from the things we need the most. Forgiveness often breaks patterns of unconscious behavior. When you make the choice to forgive, true freedom comes from within. Your willingness to forgive begins your healing process.

You can forgive your past, your inconsistencies, your choices, your enemies, your treatments that didn't work, your doctors, and your clinicians. Once you do, you can come back to that place where you can live with peace in your heart and experience true healing.

## The Transformation of Tapping

Releasing negative emotions and incorporating forgiveness and positive affirmations play a critical role in healing. Emotional Freedom Techniques (EFT), or tapping, is, as I mentioned earlier in this book, a form of emotional acupressure that releases negative emotions. It involves tapping your fingertips on acupuncture points while tuning into a problem and making statements about that problem. It is an incredibly effective technique when it is done responsibly. I love EFT. The purpose of the EFT and the GetSet™ Approach is to break the emotional connection to the perceived problem so it is only a memory. You no longer have to relive the experience, have it running your behavior in the background to protect you from further distress or limiting your happiness and potential. It changed my life and the lives of my clients from the moment I learned it and implemented it into my practice and healing.

I have found forgiveness to be such an important part of releasing negative emotions that it has become an essential part of my process. For example, I had a profound session with a woman who had been physically abused from the age of three and sexually abused for two years from the time she was ten. She came to me for a different issue, had never heard of tapping, and was gifted the session by a friend. The abuse issue just came up in the session as we were talking about the other issue. She had been in conventional therapy for twelve years. I asked if she would allow me to address the abuse in the tapping session. It was clear that she would be served by forgiving the man who had done this to her. When I suggested we tap about forgiveness, she said that during her twelve years of counseling she walked out of the office any time forgiveness came up in conversation with her therapist. She said she did not want to forgive the man. I explained that we could do this in a very gentle manner and that it was for her benefit, not necessarily his. She reluctantly agreed to give it a try.

We tapped for a couple of minutes about her not wanting to forgive him and then about being willing to forgive him someday. I said that he must have been a very wounded person to do this. I then directed her to say, "I forgive myself for allowing it to happen, for not knowing what to do, for not knowing how to stop it, for being afraid, for feeling ashamed, for thinking I may have deserved it, and for not telling anyone."

I stopped tapping with her and asked her how she felt about him. She said she felt so sorry for him. I was surprised at her response. She went on to say that she felt bad for this man because he obviously had been deeply messed up since he had considered it appropriate to sexually abuse a child. After just a few minutes, she had a completely different perspective on the situation. She said she felt completely free of the shame and anger. I asked if she would be willing to forgive him. She began to cry and replied that she just did.

This is just one example of what is possible. I am not suggesting that every issue can be cleared in five minutes. I have seen it happen numerous times.

From that point forward I have incorporated forgiveness into all my tapping sessions. When I added forgiveness, clients always seemed to come to a certain level of peace. I could see their fears or stress just melt from their faces. I would see their faces change from stern or troubled to peaceful and gentle. To get to a place of peace, they needed to not only forgive the other person for any role they felt that person played in their distress, but they also needed to forgive themselves so they could reach that necessary level of self-love and then could extend that love out into the world, to other people, and even to the people they felt hurt them or wronged them in some way.

There is always someone to forgive. It does not have to stem from a dramatic abuse situation. It may simply be that someone said, "You laugh like a girl" or "You have terrible taste in clothes." At some level, simple comments can hurt. For the most part, we simply let these things go. If you are still remembering specific comments twenty years later, chances are you have not let them go. Forgiveness will always help. In that case, it may simply be that you need to forgive yourself for holding on to it for so long.

Forgiveness works when you add it to the process. It makes healing more effective. As a scientist, I was always looking for a better way, always making sense of what I saw before me. Another thing I found with tapping was that at times people would revert to having issues with a negative emotion after releasing one. It is common for other emotional issues to come to the surface as you release one. We follow a trail to get to the core issues. I began to notice that when I added positive affirmations to tapping sessions, they became instantly more effective.

I began to test this out in my tapping sessions. I would have my clients rate the intensity of their emotion before starting and after tapping with the traditional EFT protocol. I then took a step focusing on forgiveness and had them assess their emotional intensity. Their intensity rating almost always improved. Then I would incorporate positive integration to the process and have them assess their emotional intensity. The results were phenomenal.

I developed the GetSet™ (Global Emotional Tapping Scripts and Energy Therapies) Approach after a conversation with EFT founder Gary Craig. It is simply an evolution of EFT. I have taken the foundational steps of EFT and added to it. Forgiving and positive integration are very important steps of the healing process and key components to the GetSet™ Approach. It is not part of the traditional EFT process. I believe adding these two steps have improved and elevated EFT.

Traditional EFT does not endorse the use of scripts. GetSet™ is a script-based system whereby I carefully craft each script to include forgiveness of one's self and others involved and a positive integration step. It is also a technique that people can easily learn to apply themselves. EFT has transformed thousands of lives. Many of my tapping clients say they notice significant results after just one session. Many of them reported they had struggled for decades and have even been in traditional therapy or on medication without such relief. In fact, traditional medicine has become much more accepting of tapping over the past few years, and numerous doctors have incorporated it into their practices, but it may never gain widespread acceptance in the mainstream. To discount or discredit such a technique without experiencing it because it has not been studied well enough or because we can't fully grasp how it works is a disservice to humanity.

Attitude, gratitude, and forgiveness are essential to healing. How much love, understanding, and forgiveness do you give yourself? You can't offer those to others if you don't give them to yourself. EFT and GetSet™ Tapping are tools to help you unlock these valuable pathways to your heart and soul.

## Gratitude

It's easy to focus on all the things that are going wrong, but healthy people make a conscious effort to work on appreciating the things in their lives that are going right. No matter how small it might be, focus on what is going right in your life right now. Make it a priority to practice gratitude.

Consider everything for which you are grateful. Believe in miracles. Look for bits of joy in any given moment. Do more of what you are passionate about, because there's tremendous healing power in that. Be grateful in advance for the great healing, abilities, and power that exist within you. Be grateful for the healing that is occurring in your body right now. Be grateful for the perfection for which your body functions.

One way I do this is through the use of a gratitude journal. I simply use a composition notebook and periodically pick it up and list those things for which I am grateful. When my kids were much younger, we would do a family project leading up to Thanksgiving. We would start a new gratitude book, and the whole family would participate. We kept it on the kitchen counter and encouraged everyone to add to it whenever they felt inspired to do so.

Would you be interested in starting a gratitude journal? If so, I encourage you to get very specific. List all the little things. You will never run out of things to add to your list. Be creative.

Here are just a few ideas about some things you might list in your journal:

- *Each person that is special to you or who has influenced your life in some way.*
- *List people that you don't necessarily like, but find something you are grateful for in each of them. If you*

*can't find anything nice to say, you might say you are grateful for them because they have taught you not to treat others as they have treated you, and therefore have made you a kinder or more compassionate person.*

- *Aspects of your health or body that you appreciate. You might list your heart for pumping oxygen through your body and keeping you alive, your muscles for making you feel fit, your hair for protecting your head from sunburn, your liver for detoxifying your body, your kidneys for filtering your blood, and immune system for fighting off disease like a warrior.*
- *If you have something going wrong, think about a way to spin it so you can be grateful for what is good. For instance, if you feel your eyesight is getting worse and you need to start wearing glasses, you might consider listing your eyes for being able to see all the beauty in life and for making your life so much easier. Perhaps you only need glasses while you read or while you drive. Be grateful that you can see well enough to get around your house without glasses. List some things that you can do with your vision that perhaps someone who is completely blind cannot do.*
- *The wonderful experiences that you have had.*
- *List the bad experiences you have had and list something you took away from the experience that has somehow added to your life.*
- *Your job or business. Your financial assets. Your ability to acquire what you need.*

- *The people who have crossed your path today. List the stranger who let you turn in front of them in traffic, who held the door open for you, or smiled at you in the parking lot. It is a much more powerful practice than focusing on the person who cut you off in traffic, let the door slam in your face, or gave you a dirty look. You will begin to notice more and more nice people and pleasant experiences and attract more of them into your life.*
- *Your physical stuff such as your home, electricity, car, clothing, tools, dishes, photographs, computer, telephone, and anything else that adds to your life. Get creative and have fun with this one. I remember once being at a Jack Canfield event, and he had us take a short break to appreciate everything we encountered during the break. Well, while in the restroom, I began to appreciate indoor plumbing and toilet paper. I thought for a moment about how much more complicated life would be if we didn't have toilet paper and would have to use leaves or cloth that had to be laundered or pages out of an old telephone book. Think about how different life might be without something. Suddenly you can become very grateful for things like toilet paper, toothpicks, and paperclips.*
- *Public places such as restaurants, stores, and farmers markets that make your life easier. Remember all the workers who keep those places working.*
- *The transportation systems that add to the conveniences in your life.*

- *Your pets.*
- *Your experiences.*
- *Music and entertainment sources and venues.*
- *Everything in nature. You might list trees for providing shade and oxygen, birds, butterflies, bees, worms, mountains, the oceans, rivers, and rain.*
- *Water, indoor plumbing, water filtration.*
- *Your delicious and nutritious food. Fresh fruits and vegetables. Your special treats.*

These are just a few examples of the tremendous amount of things for which you can be grateful. Supplement this list with your own specific areas of gratitude. Your list should be vast. No addition is too small. Gratitude is a powerful tool that can be used for healing both the mind and body. Be creative. Get a journal and start listing. The more we focus on gratitude, the more life gives us to be grateful for.

## Open Your Heart and Let Love Be Your Guide

Love and joy have the power to heal. We will not find the way to our heart with just our thoughts. Our minds are not the path to consciousness. Our minds are logical. Our hearts are creative. Get centered in your heart and come from that place. Come from a place of acceptance and joy. If you believe all of creation comes from love, it makes sense to understand the significance of love on nurturing life, health, and healing. That source of love is a perfect creative force.

It is also the perfect healing force.

We will find different answers if we listen with our hearts instead of our minds. The mind assesses the situation, makes judgments and predictions based on our programming, experiences, and knowledge. The mind filters out much of the information we get. When you open up and listen with your heart, it completely expands the possibilities. Seek answers with your heart and not your mind. Do so from a place of love and not fear.

Here are some questions to ask yourself while you take a moment to be still and listen to your heart:

- *Why do I want to be healthy?*
- *How can I best stay healthy?*
- *What practice can I incorporate into my life right now to give me more vibrant health?*
- *Why do I want to heal this problem?*
- *What will I do with my life when I am healed?*
- *How will I give back or be of service?*
- *How will I use my gifts, abilities, or personality for the good of others?*
- *How can I more clearly identify and fulfill my life's purpose?*

When you have an illness or physical or emotional pain, you can overcome it with a greater purpose. I believe you can also stay healthier when you live more purposefully. Love is the greatest gift. We all need to love ourselves more, all the time, every day. Through self-love we can love others. Love heals. As we heal and raise our vibration, we contribute to the well-being of others. This is a fundamental aspect of collective consciousness.

## Miracles

Many documented cases of healing have defied scientific and medical explanation. We perceive miracles as mystical and often unreachable. We often believe that they only happen to a select few. A miracle is when the forces of nature bend a little just for you. They happen in your favor, even though you may not notice them at the time. The universe is always providing the people, experiences, and resources that we need.

We cannot explain, describe, or define how miracles work. They cannot be measured, just as science can't measure a prayer and the impact it will have on someone else. They often remain a mystery and beyond our comprehension. It is a miracle when we don't understand how something might happen. It is open to our interpretation. If we fully understood it, we would no longer call it a miracle. Once the laws of nature or science can explain a miracle, it is no longer considered a miracle.

C.S. Lewis said, "Miracles do not, in fact, break the laws of nature." They are the natural way life works. Everything about our bodies and lives is a miracle. We don't need science to define how miracles work. Miracles come from

God and are more likely to happen than not. Miracles are not as mystical as we think. Life is always conspiring for us.

The truth is we make our own miracles. Healing is a miracle that is a result of proactive purpose. We can perceive our lives with doubt or with the faith that miracles will occur. Miracles happen when we are in alignment. We have to align our thoughts and beliefs with the fact that miracles are possible. We can then realize that they are probable, and we can even expect them. Be more committed to the possibility of a miracle and healing than to the "reality" of the problem or illness. As we let go of the need for proof, miracles reveal themselves to us.

Miracles are always available to us. We must open and call in the higher power for our highest good and the good of all. Pray or ask for a miracle, for help, for answers, and for healing. Be open to receiving them. Many of us feel we are not worthy of a miracle. In reality, we are all worthy of receiving miracles and they are happening for us even when we don't notice.

Make active decisions to welcome miracles. All of life is intended to be a miracle. See the wonder in it. Allow the miracles to occur and be willing to recognize and embrace them. Take any form of action toward the outcome you seek.

Expect miracles. A miracle doesn't have the same impact if no one notices it or appreciates it. Don't put conditions on or judge the miracle, just ask for it and allow it to unfold. Know that all the answers we need are already here. Believe the miracle has already happened, and feel it fully throughout your body. Imagine how it feels once the miracle has happened. As humans, we can't fully appreciate how truly magnificent we are.

If you don't have or get an answer right away, it is okay. Trust that the answer will come. Open your heart and allow the answers to come to you. Be ready to recognize and receive them. Seek that which speaks to your heart.

Look for a sign of an intervention. Being full of wonder welcomes miracles. You will find things occurring that feel unexplainable. This will often leave you in awe. You can't explain how it could have happened without some sort of spiritual intervention that is a result of some action from a higher order. It defies logic, and we can't always put it into perspective. When we believe in miracles, we elevate these laws and the miracle no longer seems inexplicable because we feel we have some vague way to describe it even when we don't know how it happens.

You will often find strange, meaningful serendipities occurring. I have heard a coincidence defined as a co-incident with God. It feels as if things come together in an almost creepy, yet joyful manner, and it brings a little smile to your face because it seems very profound, but you just don't understand how it could have happened. Sometimes you will feel a little nudge in the direction that you need to go. Do not ignore these nudges. You may get a gut feeling or even hear your inner voice.

There is always a purpose to every event in your life. No exceptions. As paths open up, we realize that something deeper and unexplainable is happening.

Nick Vujicic said, "I know for certain that God does not make mistakes, but he does make miracles. I am one. You are too." If you do not know of Nick, I would suggest you watch one of his inspiring online videos.

Albert Einstein once said, "There are only two ways to live your life. One is as though nothing is a miracle. The other is as though everything is a miracle." It is up to you to decide whether miracles are occurring around you every day. Choose wisely, because either way, you are correct.

## Ask and Be Open to Receive

The Bible says, "Ask, and it shall be given you; seek, and ye shall find; knock, and it shall be opened unto you." This has been proven to me over and over throughout the course of my life. The problem is, most of us never ask. If we do, we don't notice the answers. We don't trust our gut feelings when the solutions come to us. We don't take action on what is given to us. The truth is, the answers are longing to be received.

Ask for miracles. Ask for healing. Ask for abundant health. Ask that you will know your greatness. Ask for what you need. Ask for answers. Ask that you will be shown the way. Ask that you will easily recognize the answers.

Be proactive with your questions. Instead of asking "Why me?," ask, "What can I do about this?" Listen for the answers from the perspective of your question. The miracles are the answers that show up if you are willing to receive them. Most of us never ask. We leave everything up to fate or chance.

We pray for answers but don't always recognize them. We want miracles but don't notice them when they occur. Be open to receiving the wisdom. We must open our hearts and minds. We all have an inner guidance system. It's a matter of whether we can quiet our minds enough to hear it and if we have the faith to trust it. We don't need to force an answer. Let the answer come to you.

Learn to listen and trust your inner guidance. Pay attention to what speaks to you. Look for signs and symbols that are meaningful to you. When you feel a higher level of knowing that you can't explain, trust it. When you resonate with an idea, take action. When something just feels right, makes sense to you, or you feel intrigued by it, make note. Be silent. Be still and listen. It is not that the answer is not being provided, but that we have not developed the capacity to hear.

Some of us leave our healing up to someone else, and some obsess about the details and work hard to come up with a logical solution. While both of those may be working for us in the short term, we are often presented with the answers we need if we are willing to listen. We seek answers outside of ourselves when most often they are within. Take an introspective approach. Healing comes from within. It does not come from outside us.

My son has a tattoo that reads, "A man travels the world in search of what he needs, and returns home to find it." What I found in my journey of searching outside and finding my own cures is that the most important journey we take is the one within. All of the answers we need are within us. Trust that the universe will deliver exactly what you need.

The body always knows what to do to heal itself. If it is not healing, there is something we are doing that is preventing that process. For example, we might be depriving it of some nutrients, exposing it to too many dietary toxins, environmental toxins or conditions, depriving it of rest, or causing too much chaos in the form of emotional turmoil and stress.

Or perhaps we are asking the wrong question. I help people evaluate their lives with a discerning eye to determine what can be causing disruption in their bodies. It is all about asking the proper questions. Open yourself to the possibilities of healing and pray or ask for whatever you need to heal to show up. If you ask the question, you will draw the answer to you. Be open to recognizing the messages you will receive because they will come. If you recall, I asked and received a message about the smart meter while I was in the midst of a serious health crisis. I truly believe I would not have survived if I had not listened to that message. I would not have investigated or reduced my RF exposure and would have stayed in bed with my cell phone and cordless phone by my side. If you have trouble interpreting the message you get, ask a friend for help.

Ask that what you truly need to transform the illness or distress will be provided and that the best modality will be provided to you. You can ask in the form of prayer or use your owns spiritual insights and directly access the wisdom of your soul or higher self. Prayer is a form of vibration, and when you align your prayers with the outcome you seek, you are more likely to experience what you are asking for.

Everything you need will come to you. I am hopeful that you were led to this book for a reason and that you will find the missing piece of the puzzle that you need to turn your health around or to maintain your good health.

I had been studying natural health for several years. I knew it was time for me to play a bigger role in the world. My fears were holding me back. I wasn't ready to take the leap of faith that would allow me to have a bigger impact and reach the people that I might help. I had a terrifying fear of public speaking. I asked the universe for help. I did not know how to handle it other than to avoid public speaking altogether.

While attending a workshop, a friend and I decided to get some fresh air and venture out into a snowstorm to find a restaurant to eat lunch. As we approached the restaurant, a man and woman were ahead. The man held the door open for us. As we walked into the restaurant, the hostess asked if we were seeking a table for four. The man said, "Yes," laughed, and turned to us and asked if we were okay with that. We accepted his offer. We had a meaningful conversation over lunch and connected instantly. As fate would have it, the man became a mentor and one of my dearest friends. We attended many conferences together and explored numerous holistic modalities and life mysteries. He taught me EFT and Be Set Free Fast. Those modalities cleared my fear of public speaking instantly. The universe came through and not only provided me with the knowledge to tackle my fear but took it away completely in just minutes. It was all because I asked for help and said "yes" in a moment that life was giving me what I needed.

Many people need help or are desperately seeking answers to their challenges. I have many tools and insights that can help. Just as the universe has put many amazing people in my path that helped me, I turned it over to the universe to bring us together. Miracles began to happen. I have people tell me all the time they were guided to me in the strangest ways; one couple was even referred to me by someone atop Mount Kilimanjaro.

## Trust Your Gut

In the end, mindset, miracles, and the spiritual nature of healing are all predominately based on your ability to listen to and trust your gut. A final example will help you better understand just how. In his early teens, my son developed severe allergic reactions. One of the modalities that I use showed that he was sensitive to a number of food and chemical ingredients. With each reaction he had, we critically reviewed his dietary consumption. We figured out that he would go into anaphylactic shock if he consumed monosodium glutamate (MSG) and then exercised within a window of three to five hours. He could consume something with MSG if he wasn't going to get any physical exercise after. He could also eat food containing MSG after he exercised without any noticeable reaction. There was no doubt for any of us that it was an exercise-induced anaphylaxis and was directly related to consuming MSG. His pediatrician agreed that his condition was life threatening and prescribed antihistamines, histamine blockers, and an injectable form of epinephrine.

During a workout or run, his hands would begin to itch and within a few minutes he would start to swell. During a reaction the only place he wanted to be was in the shower. His blood pressure would drop abruptly as he swelled up. He would have to sit on the shower floor so he would not fall over. The water running over him, dye-free antihistamines, and homeopathic remedies were the only things that brought him relief.

Some would think it is irrational or neglectful not to take your child to the emergency room when he or she is having an anaphylactic reaction. In my case, I was taking a huge risk when he was going into this state. I knew at a core level that he didn't have much time and could actually die in transport. At times, the reaction came on so quickly we knew there would be no time to wait for an ambulance. On three occasions I stood on the other side of the shower curtain with a knife and a hard plastic tube knowing that at any second I might be forced to cut a tracheotomy in my son's throat to keep him alive. He was so hypersensitive to any chemicals that his gut strongly told him not to go to the emergency room. He pleaded with me not to call 911. He told me that he knew he would die if they injected him with anything. He had a very strong gut reaction to taking the epinephrine injection, and he pleaded with me anytime I offered to give it to him. It was terrifying for all of us. I trusted him. He knew his body better than anyone.

I did not take this choice lightly. I knew I would have to take responsibility if I didn't bring him in for treatment and he died. I could have even potentially faced criminal charges of neglect or endangerment. But at a soul level, I knew I had to trust him. I realized his gut was so strongly telling him not to take the intervention to the next step. I had to trust my own gut about his strong conviction that medical intervention would be catastrophic. I had to consider that if I gave him the shot, called the paramedics, or took him to the emergency room, he could die.

Who really knows if my son would have had a negative reaction or died had we injected him with the epinephrine emergency kit? What if a massive dose of steroids would have killed him? The truth is we don't know.

Because his reaction was so severe, I wanted it documented by a specialist. We proceeded to go to a highly respected allergist. We told the allergist that my son had this severe reaction to MSG, and she told us that it was impossible to have an allergy to a chemical. She said whatever he was eating was just a coincidence and that he had exercise-induced anaphylaxis. She suggested my son give up sports. My son had been in sports since he was in preschool, and this was not an option. Our goal was to find a way to keep him in sports and prevent these reactions.

We learned to manage the reaction without seeking medical intervention. I am not suggesting that anyone else do this. I am simply sharing this to tell you how we handled this scenario and that it worked for us. He trusted his gut above all else. We figured out what caused the reaction, we figured out the best way to manage it if he inadvertently ingested MSG, and he learned how to read labels. We put our faith in our guts. My son survived a dozen episodes of anaphylaxis over the years without steroids or epinephrine injections.

The point of this story is to listen to your doctor, but also trust yourself. Your doctor does not know you better than you know yourself. Hear what he or she says, and weigh your options. Your goal is to seek information from your doctor. Your best option might be to do exactly as your doctor tells you. Trust the feedback your body is giving you. Healing is a state of mind, a way of being. In your life, work to make healthy choices that make you feel good and remain aligned with your overall goals. Health is your most precious resource. Without it, all the money and time in the world will matter little. Treat it as such, and protect it, cherish it, and celebrate it.

# Chapter 8

# The Power of Belief

Are you ready to experience vibrant health? Do you feel worthy of doing so? Do you believe it is possible on a physical, emotional, spiritual, and energetic level? What if healing powers could be summoned with just your mindset and intention when you are an energetic match with the outcome that you want? What if healing is not as mystical as we think? What if we could enhance and support our bodies' natural ability to heal?

A number of cultures throughout the world maintain that there is an energetic force that can be directed to an outcome simply by intending it to be so. While it is not a concept that is widely accepted in traditional medicine, we often see this in action in life. This chapter will open with a discussion on intention, belief, and affirmations. The vibration of the words we speak and the thoughts we think impact our health and the outcomes in our lives. These can influence our physiology, our genetic expression, and our health.

## Belief in Healing

We have a hard time believing that which we cannot experience with our five senses. If we can't see it, touch it, or feel it, we tend to think it doesn't exist. As hard as it may be to understand, we are creating our lives with every thought we think, every belief we have, and with every action we take.

Our thoughts are often separate from the reality we experience. Our beliefs about what we are experiencing become our reality. Proverbs 23:7 states, "For as a man thinketh in his heart, so is he." I interpret this to say we become what we strongly believe about ourselves.

Ancient traditions relied upon a belief in healing, and that has been lost over time. The belief that healing has already occurred is a key element to invoke healing. There is tremendous power in maintaining a belief that a cure is not only possible but that it has already manifested itself in your life.

Have a deep faith and passion for the things you believe in and for the possibilities that exist. Healing begins when we intend to heal. Intention shapes our reality. Healing manifests when we align our beliefs, feelings, and actions with our intention. You cannot believe anything that you don't accept as being true or possible. We create our own limitations with our beliefs or lack thereof. In reality, our thoughts contribute to either disease or to healing.

## Challenge Your Programming

We have all been conditioned by our past. Conditioning tells us what is possible and what is not. A belief is something we think is true through our interpretation of our programming. If you believe you can't be healed as a result of your conditioning, you probably won't be healed. You can't heal with the same mindset and circumstances that caused the dis-ease.

Henry Ford said, "Whether you think you can, or you think you can't, either way you are correct." Our families and society influence our belief systems. Your family conditions you to settle or to excel. I have noticed a trend in my clients that have been conditioned to "be realistic." "Reality" has often stopped them from healing and from dreaming big.

Illusions have the same power as truths. We often cling to false beliefs. Sometimes we need to face the very things that go against our beliefs. We need to challenge our programming and decide what is true for us.

When I was a child, my elementary school started a band program. Instruments were put on display there so we could choose the one we wanted to play. The trombone fascinated me. When I met with the band director and told him I wanted to play it, he laughed and said trombones were for boys and that girls don't play the trombone. He suggested I select a different instrument. There was nothing else I wanted to play. I had set my hopes on the trombone. I walked out of the office feeling sad and defeated. I gave up my dream of playing the trombone because someone told me it wasn't normal for a girl to want to play it. While I no longer have an interest in this instrument, I have learned valuable lessons from that little girl who gave up and didn't stand up for what she wanted. It took many years, but I eventually learned not to allow myself to be limited by someone else's opinion or reality about what is possible.

Luckily, I was blessed with a family that always encouraged me to be all that I could. As a result, I chose to experience life as being full of possibilities. People have often told me they saw my life as being full of exciting adventures and experiences. In my teens and twenties, friends and colleagues said I should write a book about my experiences. I never really understood why my life seemed more exciting to them than their own. It was not until recently that I realized the way I experienced life was a result of choosing to be curious and open to possibilities. I set a subconscious intention to be full of wonder and surrounded by supercool people. Even though it was not intentional, I expected it and it became my reality.

## Intention Changes Your Experience

The good news is that you can change your intention for your life at any point. You do not have to be restricted by societal pressures. You can change your programming simply by consciously deciding to do so. It does not take a lot of time or effort.

You have more control than you might realize. Consider the possibilities your life would hold if you let go of your limitations. If there was just one thing from this book that you could integrate into your life, I believe the most important one would be the realization of the power you have within you to be all that you were created to be simply by believing it is possible and by choosing to take even a small amount of action toward it.

This is not just about being positive. A positive mindset is helpful. Intention and belief are much more powerful than attitude. We can fake an attitude. We can be positive without actually believing it. We can believe it will all work out without having a specific intention for what that will look like in the end.

We don't need science to defend how this all works. Science will never fully understand how or why this works. Science can't measure how someone can say a prayer for another person who is across the country and that person receives the prayer or miracle or is affected in some way.

Marianne Williamson once said that we can heal the body with the mind, but we cannot heal the mind with the body. Your thoughts can contribute to disease. The mind can also prevent and reverse disease. It has tremendous power over the physical experience. When you align your mindset with healing, your body will follow. When you change your perception, you change your experience and how you live. The universe will give you miracles to the extent that you believe they are possible. Intention gives you a vision for life. When you set an intention, you not only believe it is possible, but you make a decision to expect a specific outcome.

Essentially the placebo effect is reflective of this. Studies have proven the power of this effect. This means that someone heals because they believe they will heal. They think they are given the treatment when in fact they are given a sugar pill. It is scientifically measurable. Results are not just by chance. Changes in emotional states, beliefs, and human consciousness affect outcomes and cause changes in the physical world.

It is the influence of the belief that something will or will not affect the outcome. If you give the body what it needs and take away what is harming it, then you will heal. I am not saying that we are capable of living forever. There is a natural order to life, and it has a time frame. When our time is up, there is nothing we can do to change that. However, we have much more control than we believe over our quality of life and level of health. Einstein said, "Imagination is more important than knowledge." Contemplate the idea that we have more influence on the world than the world has on us.

My friend is a teacher and conducted a classroom experiment based on the work of Dr. Masaru Emoto. She wanted to illustrate the power of words, thoughts, and intentions to her students. She boiled a pot of white rice and separated the rice into two clean mason jars. She labeled one jar "love" and the other jar "hate." Over the course of several weeks, she kept the jars in a prominent location in her classroom. The students were instructed to send positive thoughts and feelings to the jar labeled "love" and negative thoughts and feelings to the jar labeled "hate." Months later, my friend showed me the jars. The rice in the jar receiving positive thoughts was white and fluffy and looked good enough to eat. The rice in the jar receiving negative thoughts was not recognizable. It had lost its form and looked like black paste. This shows the power of intention and the influence it has over biology.

Your thoughts, emotions, and beliefs affect your cells. Your cells chemically process your thoughts and beliefs. Believe that your body is perfect the way it is. Trust the inner wisdom of your body to restore balance and health in your body.

Every thought shapes our reality. Don't put your thoughts on the things you don't want. Put or direct your thoughts and attention on the outcome you want. Do not focus on the problem. Focus on finding the solution.

Create the vision of what you want. Do no focus on what is, but on what might be. Visualize yourself free of the problem. Feel what it would be like to be free of the problem or condition. Feel the vibrancy in your body. Feel the joy, excitement, and enthusiasm. Think about all the possibilities of all the things you will be able to do when this perceived problem is no longer holding you back. Intend that it is done. It is that simple.

## Take One Small Step at a Time

From the time I was a little girl, I wanted to save the world. I wanted to make it a better, safer, more peaceful place.

Injustices troubled me deeply. I didn't know how I would save the world, I just felt it was my responsibility and I wanted to do it. I was young and had not yet been conditioned to believe I had limits. Eventually, I realized it was too big a job for one person. The level of responsibility was paralyzing. Then I realized I could do it one person at a time. When you have a big goal or dream that is too big for your mind, start by taking one small step. Break it down, and view it from another perspective.

I was recently coaching a practitioner who was troubled by lack of product sales. I shared the following story with him: I had spent a year writing a book, a year working with the publisher, and thousands of dollars. I make about one dollar per book sold. On the day the book launched, I sold forty-three copies. I told a friend that I was a bit discouraged and embarrassed by the low number. He said that my book had the power to change lives and if I helped forty-three people improve their lives, it was all worth it. His point was well taken. I do believe my books have the potential to transform lives or I wouldn't have invested years of my life writing them. I learned that I needed to let go of my attachment to the number and focus on the impact my work was having.

As I shared this story with my coaching client, I suggested he turn it over to the universe and believe that his products get into the hands of everyone who needs them and is ready to hear the information he has to offer. I advised him to focus on the impact rather than the numbers. By focusing on impacting a huge number of people rather than having a huge sales figures, he grew his sales. More importantly, he reached more people with his work. I have shared this story many times and gotten lots of positive feedback. It helps to get the mind out of the way and make a big goal more manageable.

I recommend you take small steps with the suggestions I provide in this book. It is much easier to get results when you don't feel overwhelmed with a gigantic task or changing your whole life. Set an intention and take one small action step toward that intention. Focus on the benefits and impact as if you have already achieved success.

**Life Takes Care of the Details**

The following story illustrates the power of intention: I had been looking to purchase a book for children on EFT, but couldn't find any. Turns out there weren't any at that time. Then I began to think that I should write it, but I quickly dismissed this idea because I didn't know the first thing about how to write or publish a book. I heard Jack Canfield talk about intention. He suggested we think of something that was not likely to happen and set an intention and create an affirmation about that intention. He said to make it something that was so unlikely that we would know for certain that this process worked. I went blank. I could not think of anything. This children's book popped in and out of my head, but I continued to dismiss it because I really didn't have an interest in being the one to do it.

Feeling the pressure to write an affirmation right there on the spot in fear that I may not go back to the exercise, I reluctantly wrote this affirmation: "I am happy and grateful now that I have successfully written and published my children's tapping book and it gets to everyone around the world that will benefit from it."

On my flight home, I was looking over my notes and saw my affirmation. I started to make a list of the things that might go into a book like this. I could not stop. I wrote for the duration of the three-hour flight. I began to wonder if I could in fact write a book. I began to believe in the possibility. The month that followed was full of amazing synchronicities. Not only did I write the entire book, I found my neighbor was an editor and made time to edit the book, I found a way to publish the book, and I asked someone I highly respected who knew tapping and had a passion for working with kids to write the foreword. Within a year, *Tap into Joy* was published in English and in Japanese, and I began receiving e-mails from people all over the world thanking me for writing it.

The point of this story is that when we are in alignment with our purpose and intentionally living life, life takes care of all the details in a way that transcends human understanding. I had no idea how all those details fell into place, but they did. The more I believed it, the more it became my reality. I started to see how critical this was to healing. I began to look back over the years on why some clients had healed and others had not.

## More Reasons People Don't Heal

People don't heal as quickly as they can because they don't believe it can happen. They leave it up to chance. They wait to see what happens with their body. They sit back and wait for each doctor's visit and each test result to come in. They limit the possibilities to what is "realistic" based on their prognosis or what science can predict.

Wanting something, hoping for, wishing for, or relying on chance for something is not enough. Praying for an outcome is not enough. God gives us free will and expects us to act and work toward what we desire. Allow the healing power of your body to manifest healing, harmony, and perfect health. Know that your body strives to be well and in balance.

You can do it. I have done it. No one showed me how. To me, it seemed to have occurred by chance. I didn't understand how it happened until I reverse engineered what I had done in each case after the fact. I now know it was all orchestrated by God to help me figure out my purpose. Sharing insights from my story of healing and that of others is my purpose right now as I understand it.

Instead of asking, "Why me?," ask yourself, "Why did this happen for me? What is it teaching me? What skills have I developed in the process? How can I use these skills to help others? Who can I help? How can I serve?" If you listen closely, you will come up with an answer. It may not be in the form of words. It may be a gut feeling or an image. Pay attention. You can also view other circumstances of your experiences through this lens.

### Shifting Paradigms

A paradigm is simply a pattern of beliefs that creates your reality. Mine has been challenged several times. It has also completely shifted as a result of learning from my life experiences and deeply exploring my truth.

Jim Walters said, "The dilemma of our existence is choosing what to believe." What do you believe about your health and the experiences of your life? We have free choice to make our own decisions about our health based on our beliefs and what we feel is best for ourselves and our families.

As an empathetic person, many times I have been moved to tears by a story a client shared with me. I have empathized with them for their prognosis while maintaining hope that I could lead them to an answer they needed in order to heal. I have learned that we achieve better results when I believe they have already healed. Some may argue that this is the placebo effect. In essence, it is.

People who come to me have a couple of things in common. Even if they are skeptical, they believe there is a chance they will find some new piece of information or direction and they are willing to explore it. This is a powerful place to be, and I believe this is the basis of their results. When I go into a session with a client, I pray for guidance to help him or her and in gratitude for his or her health and well-being. I ask that I will be used to the highest level of my soul's calling. I complete my query with, "and so it is, it is done."

## The Influence of a Diagnosis

A diagnosis has tremendous power. Once we accept a diagnosis, it often becomes part of our identity. When we feel that life has thrown us a curveball, or served us an injustice, we often lose hope. It is easy to give up hope when we feel defeated and victimized. There is a Buddhist principle which teaches that all suffering comes from attachment. We often lose ourselves in that diagnosis. We become attached to the diagnosis. We get caught up in the fear and the prognosis. When we believe we are a victim, we feel that we must be taken care of. We give up our power. We suffer through the time that passes between each doctor's visit and diagnostic test. The diagnosis becomes our reality.

When you take on the disease as part of your identity, you will have a very hard time healing. You don't have to accept a diagnosis. Don't let a disease or disorder define you. Never give up hope. Be a participant in your health. Be present in your life. Consider the work that you are doing as part of your healthcare, rather than dis-ease care. We must not nurture the illness, but nurture the healing. Accept and honor where you are right now.

Release any stress and toxic emotions such as blame or guilt. Our judgments of ourselves or others can block our progress. Stress suppresses our immune system. It does not serve us to focus on the stress and the fear of the unknown. Know that you have done the best you could up until this point. It is normal to have some fears and negative thoughts. Acknowledging your feelings is the first step toward working through them and getting to a place of empowerment.

Believing a diagnosis or prognosis is aligning your intention with the current state. You do not want to stay in that state. Many doctors admit that a patient's symptoms and illness increase once a diagnosis is given. This phenomenon is known as the nocebo effect. If you expect to experience declining health or negative side effects, you often will. Like the placebo effect, the nocebo effect is a self-fulfilling prophecy. In either case, you experience results based on your belief about your current state or fears about your future state of health.

There are key factors to consider. I believe the way you accept or believe in a diagnosis will affect your outcome more than just relying on the odds of either treating or not treating a condition. Through my work in a funeral home, I have heard many families say their loved one was given so many months to live and they died in exactly that time frame. I have come to understand that a patient's life expectancy is heavily influenced by their expectations and belief about their prognosis.

Having hope gives us much more power than we realize. Accepting a diagnosis and a gloomy prognosis takes away much of our power. Summon all the courage you can, and take back your power. Hope equals possibility. Possibility equals belief in an anticipated outcome.

This doesn't just apply to disease or health issues. It is applicable to any area of your life. It holds true for our relationships, our finances, our jobs, and our confidence to step boldly into life. I often see people who are struggling to find out what is wrong with them. Instead of looking for the cause, they look for a diagnosis. I often tell them that, if they continue this practice, they will eventually find something to be diagnosed with. If you keep going for X-rays and CT scans or trying multiple drugs and therapies, you are probably more likely to develop a problem. Drugs may tame a symptom but inevitably impair other functions and processes in the body. There are risks associated with some diagnostic procedures. We explored some of these in Chapter 3. Simply going through the testing looking for something wrong affirms your belief that there is something wrong and puts you in a position to actually experience the disease.

It is human nature to want to know what is going on in our bodies. Never ignore a symptom. Focus on why it is happening rather than on the problem or diagnosis. It is a matter of tweaking your mindset to be proactive.

Illness is a process. We are conditioned to be realistic. We adapt to the current state. This conditioning causes us to have expectations about the outcome. What have you been conditioned to believe about this diagnosis or about the one who has given you the diagnosis?

What we focus our attention on expands. When we stay focused on the illness, symptoms, or the diagnosis, we reinforce the thoughts and subconscious beliefs that created the illness and keep it persisting. You may not want to identify or label it.

I recently saw a billboard that said one in five teenagers uses drugs. My initial thought was that this was a lot of kids using drugs. Then I realized that "one in five" means four in five or 80 percent of teenagers don't. If we focus on the 80 percent of teens who don't, and if teens focus on the 80 percent who don't, maybe they will be less likely to use drugs. I am not suggesting we ignore the drug problem or don't offer support to those in need.

If I were a susceptible teen who was influenced by peer pressure and thought many kids did drugs, I might be more apt to take that path and join the crowd. On the other hand, if I were presented with the fact that most teens live drug-free and find ways to cope and manage their pressures in healthy ways, I would be more likely to seek those ways. What we put our attention on grows. Wouldn't we rather grow the number of teens who don't use drugs than the number of teens who do?

Not wanting certain problems, diseases, or symptoms keeps your attention on the problem. If you keep your attention on wishing the problem away, you keep your attention on the problem. Focus on what you want. Focus on vibrant health.

During the radiofrequency crisis that I discussed in Chapter 5, I sought help from doctors to figure out what was causing the problems, but they had no way of figuring it out. I did not want to overidentify with my physical body. I did not want to become the state of dis-ease in my body. I opted not to receive any definitive diagnosis and did not focus on identifying with the disease.

Over the course of many months, my family watched me go from a vibrant, energetic woman to a depleted, frail woman who could barely function. My son asked, "Mom, do you have cancer?" I replied, "It doesn't matter." I explained that I was not hiding a diagnosis from anyone. I knew that something was poisoning me and the only thing that would serve me was to find the cause. Treating the disease was not part of my plan.

I did not openly share my condition while I was in the

midst of it. I did not want others focused on my failing health. I did not want to be influenced by the energetic effect of other people's fears, sympathy, judgments, or worries. Those practices would not support my healing or serve them in any way.

I put all of my energy into focusing on finding the cause. In the end, I found the cause and my answers did not come from conventional sources. In a moment of prayerful meditation, I received the message about my smart meter. My decision to focus my efforts on the cause served me much better than seeking a label and a treatment for it.

Some of us pray for healing but don't always believe it is possible. We don't always believe we are worthy of it. Sometimes we want to heal but push healing away by believing that it is not likely, the odds are against us, or because we get a secondary benefit from being sick. We might also have so much fear around the illness that we cannot come into alignment energetically with the end result of being healed. When we live from a place of fear, we see our circumstances as threatening and everything seems to have conditions attached.

Often, patients are put on antidepressants when traditional medicine can't reach a diagnosis or when a patient has emotional challenges. It is normal to feel frustration, sadness, and fear when you experience loss or uncertainty. In my experience, these medications numb you from experiencing life. Be sure you have the support you need when you are going through a crisis and know that medication is not the only answer. Any dose adjustment or weaning should be done under medical supervision.

I urge people to allow themselves to experience their feelings. There's great wisdom behind each of them. Think about the disease as a process or experience rather than an endpoint. It is helpful to release fear and anxiety while you are dealing with any dis-ease. It's also helpful to release some of the beliefs about why you have developed the disease in the first place. It is not as difficult or as time consuming as it may sound, and it gives you tremendous freedom. Think about what you are learning from this illness or problem. What is it teaching you about your journey here? Really sit with that question and ponder possible answers.

From the perspective of healing, I no longer believe we need to secure a diagnosis. By assigning a diagnosis, we interfere with the healing process and can influence the outcome with the nocebo effect. From the perspective of traditional medicine, being able to provide a diagnosis is considered to be one of the greatest strengths. If a diagnosis is important to you, I urge you to seek a medical evaluation. You may want to rule out a serious condition. Remember to keep your attention on finding and eliminating the cause.

### The Power of Words

Our words act as a self-fulfilling prophecy. Whether positive or negative, our bodies believe our words as affirmations.

We are creating affirmations when we refer to a dis-ease with phrases like, "I think I have . . .," "I have . . .," "My . . .," "It's in my genes . . .". In those instances, we alter our gene expression simply with our words and the energy behind them.

Be careful about your language in respect to a symptom or diagnosis. When people call it "my cancer," they take it on and it becomes part of them. When you say things like "my knee problem," "my bad shoulder," "I have diabetes," "I have three months to live," "I'm destined to have this," "It's all a part of getting older," or "It's in my genes," you are affirming this to be your reality. Your mind believes what you say. I tell people to believe that it is only a temporary condition. Find the cause of the problem on your own, with the assistance of this book, or enlist the help of someone you trust and believe in. Never give up hope. Know that there is always another way. Explore your options. Educate yourself. Make the best decision you can, and then go with it.

This disease is not yours. Do not make it yours. When I talk about a diagnosis, I am not speaking only to those with a "disease" such as cancer, asthma, or diabetes. Realize you can relate this to anything you may be going through, any symptom, pain, condition, fear, anxiety, or anything you may be concerned with. The more you talk about the disease, the more you perpetuate it. Every cell in our bodies responds energetically to every word we hear and every thought we think. Every thought and belief we create is an affirmation. It can be positive or negative. The universe hears what you say. Choose to stay healthy at all costs. Use words to affirm the outcome you want. Claim your health.

When you make a conscious decision to watch your wording, you will catch yourself "slipping." Invite your friends, family, or an accountability buddy to help you with this. Give them permission to point it out when they hear you claiming it as "my problem, condition, illness, or disorder."

If we make statements and believe we are *going to* heal, we are pushing that reality off into the future. We are saying that at some point we will heal. This is not good enough. Wanting it or hoping for it is not enough. Sometimes praying for it alone is not enough, especially if you are only asking for a result. When you want or long for perfect health, the core belief is about the lack of it. Take responsibility and do something about it. Change your belief and your wording. Give thanks for the results, turn the "how" over to a higher power, then shift your focus to finding the cause and having the health that you desire.

Words can create an excuse to do nothing. Take the word *try* for example. When you try to get to something, chances are you will not do it. When you say *try*, you let yourself off the hook if you fail. Decide if you are serious about taking some form of action. Either commit to doing it or let it go. Be in integrity with yourself over the decision that you have made. If you really want to commit to not eating chocolate at night, instead of saying "I will try not to eat chocolate at night," say "I no longer eat chocolate at night." Many of us want to exercise more than we do. Instead of saying, "I will try to get to the gym three times per week" say, "I will go to the gym on Mondays, Wednesdays, and Fridays before work." The latter sets you up to be more accountable and ensures a higher probability of following through. Watching out for this simple three-letter word will make a big difference in the outcome.

Choose your words wisely because they are powerful and can impact your health and well-being.

**The "Have to Get to" Game**

Here is a simple exercise that helps you integrate the mindful use of words. I call it the "Have to Get to" game. Take a task of which you are not fond. Instead of saying, "I have to do the dishes," say "I get to do the dishes." When you "get" to do something, it forces you to shift your focus on gratitude and to positive aspects, such as being physically capable of doing it, having running water, having a source of fuel to heat the water, having dishes and soap and space to put them. When you "have to" do something it feels like you are doomed and obligated to do it. "Have to" makes it a chore. "Get to" makes it a blessing.

Keep in mind that this is an exercise in the mindful awareness of the words you choose. It is about catching ourselves and making a better choice. Being able to easily shift your perspective is a blessing in itself and has a powerful impact. Have fun with this. It will work. When you "get to" clean up your dog's poop, you are blessed to be physically able to do it, to have a dog, to have a place for him to poop, and that he is healthy enough to eat and poop.

Instead of saying I have to go for treatment, say I get to go for treatment. Say it with unshakeable confidence that the treatment is fixing the problem. You may not believe it at first. The old saying "Fake it until you make it" works in this case.

## Affirmations Affect Reality

Positive affirmations have tremendous power. This is not just about having a positive outlook. Affirmations are statements we make about the desired outcome we want. Make statements that incorporate the outcome you want in the present tense, as if they have already occurred.

Since we learn differently, I encourage you to write your affirmation, look at it, and say it aloud when you think about it. You may wish to display the affirmation in an area where you will regularly see it in order to remind you. I often recommend putting your affirmation on your bathroom mirror. You can use a sticky note or write it directly on the mirror with a marker that will easily wash off when you want to change your affirmation. Saying your affirmation in front of a mirror is helpful to overcome any disbelief in achieving the end result. If you want to keep your affirmation confidential, you may wish to post a reminder by simply posting a colorful dot or something that will trigger you to remember to repeat and think about your affirmation.

Consider the following examples for your affirmations:

- *"I am happy and grateful now that I am healthy and vibrant."*
- *"I am happy and grateful that my body is working in perfect harmony."*
- *"I am happy and grateful because I am healed."*
- *"I am full of energy."*
- *"Everything I need is provided to me."*
- *"I am safe and healthy."*
- *"I joyfully take care of my mind and body."*
- *"I deserve abundant health."*
- *"I feel the joy of perfect health."*

You can have multiple affirmations or just one. Do what feels best to you, and realize that you can change your affirmation whenever you desire. Do not worry about how you will reach the end result. Allow the universe to provide what you need.

## Genetics—We Are Not as Predisposed as We Think

When I took genetics in college in the 1980s, we were taught that our genes determined everything and that we were powerless over them. It took me many years to undo this belief.

Conventional medicine ignores the role of energy and quantum physics in healing. Once you understand energy, you realize it has more control over biology than molecules, chemicals, hormones, or physiology. The truth is that our genes do not control us. We are not victims of our genetic code unless we believe we are powerless or somehow doomed. It is easy to change the expression of our genes. Scientific studies have proven this. Believe in the possibilities.

I have great respect for the study of epigenetics and the work of brilliant scientists such as Bruce Lipton and the late Candace Pert. Epigenetics studies how the environment controls gene activity.

Our DNA is not a death sentence. Despite the fact that genes are linked to various medical problems, we really understand so little about them. One thing is becoming increasingly obvious, and that is that our food, thoughts, beliefs, and emotions cause physiological and biochemical responses that can turn our genes on or off. Our cells analyze and respond to stimuli in their environment. When you change the way you experience life events, you change your gene expression. Our life choices, food choices, stress, and sleep patterns can also alter how our genes are expressed.

It is an injustice when people are told they have a genetic predisposition to something and then make life-altering decisions in response. There is a big difference between a gene that is linked to a disease and a gene actually causing that disease. The BRCA1 and BRCA2 genes that have been linked to breast cancer can best illustrate an example of this. Scientists agree that a very small percentage of breast cancers are caused by an inherited gene. Some women are having mastectomies after being identified as carriers of this gene because they fear getting breast cancer. I do not believe a doctor should remove any healthy body part because of fear. This speaks to greed, ignorance, or lack of integrity. It is biologically possible to suppress the expression of certain genes. Genes can be altered simply with intention, belief, and a nourishing environment. It is proven science. Studies have shown that healing intentions can have positive effects on the body.

Most experts say that less than 5 to 10 percent of genetic defects are true genetic abnormalities that as of yet cannot be altered. I believe there is a cause for each genetic issue. I do not feel they are flaws made by God. I believe they are physiological responses to some past exposure. Perhaps the great grandmother was exposed to a physical toxin or emotional trauma that altered her DNA and she passed that down to the next generations. Maybe there was a spiritual agreement you made when you came to this world to experience the deepest form of connection and unconditional love to nurture a child with a genetic disorder through life.

I recently met a woman who has an adult son with Down

syndrome. He is struggling with complications that are considered terminal, and because of the level of care he requires, he has been placed in a nursing home. His eighty-five-year-old mother drives an hour each way every day to visit him. I thanked her for her commitment to him and explained how I had just returned from doing a keynote presentation for a Down syndrome society in Canada.

I expressed how moved I was to feel the tremendous love and support of the families and the unconditional joy the Down children exhibited. I felt blessed to know this. She briefly shared some things about her fifty-year-old son. She said he was never angry or resentful, he had never heard a swear word or witnessed injustice, never judged, and never wanted or begged for anything. He was simply happy all the time. Tears welled up in my eyes as I felt her love and his unconditional love for life. What a gift to experience life from his perspective.

There are some true "genetic defects." Down syndrome is an example. There is nothing we know to do that will change the outcome genetically. We do not understand enough about it. There is a reason. We don't understand it yet and for now, it is important to recognize the gift.

I don't proclaim to have all the answers, but I do know we have more influence than we are conditioned to believe. Bruce Lipton, PhD, said, "The moment you change your perception is the moment you rewrite the chemistry of your body."

Truth is a continuous journey. We never have all the answers. Our beliefs continually evolve. In science, we are discovering new things about the human body all the time. Most of our DNA, up to 95 percent, is considered junk DNA because no one has figured out why it is there. We know the brain has more capacity than we can explain. I don't believe God makes junk and gave us anything we don't need. We simply don't understand its role. I am certain that the majority of our DNA is not just "filler." I don't claim to know its function, but I believe it has a purpose and that it is more spiritual in nature than we can imagine at this point in time.

Belief is a very powerful component of healing. Being intentional about the words you choose can impact your health and the outcome of the events in your life. When you experience any type of symptom or medical problem, remember there is always something causing it. You will experience more of what you focus on. You can keep your attention on the problems or keep your attention on the solutions. Be proactive about your health and always keep your attention on your desired outcome. Vibrant health is the goal.

In the upcoming chapters, we will discuss how self-care and spiritual practices contribute to your well-being. This includes prioritizing your needs, finding balance in your life, and seeking meaningful experiences that you feel passionate about.

# Chapter 9

# Self-Care

They say there is no care like self-care. Self-care is taking time to and focusing energy on maintaining a deep and dedicated emphasis on your own health. To take the best care of ourselves, we must recognize areas in our lives where we do a disservice to ourselves, causing unnecessary burden and stress on our bodies and minds. Once we do this, we then need to find ways to nurture ourselves back to optimal health. That is the goal of this chapter.

## Negative Programming

Society conditions us for mediocrity. Our schools, media, employers, and religious organizations teach us to follow their model, which may not be the best model for each of us. At almost all levels, society teaches us to conform to the system and participate as just one member of the herd, instead of thinking for ourselves and standing out as an individual. Taking care of yourself starts with recognizing *why* you are conditioned a certain way, how it has affected you, and then making the decision to shift those beliefs so you can be more of your true, brilliant self.

We are conditioned to think negatively. The media continuously instills fear in us by flashing constant images of what is going wrong in the world, of the dangers surrounding us, and showing us how ordinary people just like us are victimized and brutalized. Many of us are tormented by the news, yet stay fixated on watching it on a daily basis. Sadly, the news introduces a remarkable amount of negativity and propaganda into our lives. Through graphic images and visuals, we become part of the moment and then take away a clear picture of the death and despair surrounding us. It puts us in a position to manifest negative events in our own lives and remain in a state of fear and dysfunctional thought, which is counterproductive to our growth and development. The old saying goes, "If it bleeds, it leads." This is not the type of mantra we want to invite in.

Fear is a very influential emotion. It programs our instincts to do what we have to do to survive. As an example, the networks will seduce you with scares of bird flu, swine flu, Ebola outbreaks, and other diseases to sell you vaccines and treatments. A small percentage of cases may occur worldwide, and the pharmaceutical industry will then likely take credit for stopping it in its tracks. Generally, the risk of infection is not high enough to justify the attention and worry we put into it. Don't allow yourself to fall victim to the hype. You will be just as likely to die from a lightning strike or from falling into a sinkhole as you would a media-pushed illness. I have seen many people rearrange their plans because of fears of epidemic outbreaks or terror threats that did not materialize. My work gives me the opportunity to regularly travel. While I do not want to be exposed to a deadly virus or held hostage in a plane, I will not allow fear to creep in and rain on my parade, especially when that fear is unrealistic and at least statistically unjustified. Use common sense and trust your gut instincts to stay safe, but do not allow anyone to instill irrational fears in you.

There is little in the news or media that will be significant in your life in a month or two unless you create it by visualizing and worrying about it. The worst times to watch news are first thing in the morning and last thing at night, when your mind is most influenced by what you feed it.

To ensure that I do not get lost in the propaganda, I have received all my news over the past twenty-five years from public broadcasting and trusted Internet sources. I do not claim to be an expert on world events or politics because I choose to distance myself from much of it. From my perspective, the news spins it to give you one side of a story for a particular agenda, and in the end, the news brings you down and puts you in a state of anxiety when you do pay close attention to it. Be very intentional about what you choose to watch on television or what you pay attention to in the media. Select only those programs (it is no mistake that they are called programs) that are in alignment with your interests, beliefs, and values. Filter out everything else. There are unbiased sources of media, but you must seek them out. Otherwise you will be programmed with a lot of propaganda and find yourself susceptible to negative self-programming, which will carry a lasting impact on your health, mood, emotions, and overall view of the world.

## The Benefit of Being Sick

When we neglect our well-being, our bodies develop symptoms to slow us down and teach us to take better care of ourselves. In our busy lives, it is sometimes easier to push past the symptom or take a pill or other remedy and keep going than it is to identify and eliminate the cause and give our bodies the proper rest and fuel that they need.

We often create our own limitations in healing. The body is so wise that it will create problems to protect us from other problems or from facing things that are difficult for us. There is usually some benefit of being sick, staying sick, or having some symptom of sickness. It may be unpleasant and difficult to see the benefits at first, but they do exist. It may not seem like a justifiable reason to have the illness, or to tolerate the discomfort, but it is a benefit nonetheless.

At times, our bodies need support so badly that being sick or injured is the best way for us to get what we want. The benefit may be that it gets us attention or sympathy, it gets us off the hook, it delays something that is unpleasant, gives us an excuse to shut down, to rest, to become reclusive, protects us from a fear, protects us from a painful emotion, keeps us detached from an unhealthy relationship, removes us from the spotlight, or just offers us some time off. Sickness reminds us that we are human and need to take care of ourselves. Sometimes we simply need to be nurtured and loved a little bit more.

### The Victim Mindset

We play small and want to fit in. We don't want to stand out or look like we are trying to be better than everyone else. In fact, we are hiding our magnificence. We are much more magnificent than most of us can admit or give ourselves credit for. This can create a victim mindset, where we stay stuck in our comfort zone and choose not to progress through life, but at a subconscious level actually set ourselves up for catastrophic failure. Once you identify the reasons and overcome the emotional issues that keep you stuck or feeling defeated, you can move forward through the healing process and find more happiness in your life.

We all struggle with worthiness at times. There are a number of ways we can work to release this programming that has reinforced the belief that we are not worthy of experiencing more in life or that we are somehow not good enough. We have all been hurt, shamed, or beaten down in our own experiences, and it is often easier to secretly believe in these thoughts than to overcome them. It is difficult to heal and move forward when you are constantly beating yourself up or feeling stuck.

Everyone has experienced some level of grief or loss. Grief causes many people to feel victimized and to stop living to the fullest extent. Many of us have experienced a traumatic event, and our biggest fear is that we will have to go through it again. Often the trauma associated with the memory has us reliving the trauma on a regular basis. The fear of it happening again keeps us stuck and unwilling or unable to fully feel and express joy.

We have a choice to feel empowered in the face of adversity or victimized by it. Feeling and acting like a victim makes us seem hopeless and often helpless. Sometimes that feels more comfortable as we may crave downtime and compassion from others. We may at some level need nurturing. It is common to need to feel held and supported through difficult times. This is different than dwelling on an experience from the perspective of a victim's mindset. A victim mindset does not help you expand or heal. It causes you to blame someone or something outside of yourself for your illness, loss, distress, or unhappiness. It holds us back and leaves us feeling disempowered. There are better, more effective ways to nurture yourself that do not impede your advancement in life. As we act as victims, we often allow negative feelings to creep in.

Negative emotions have negative vibrations and are toxic. Take an inventory of the anger, guilt, resentment, sadness, or stress you are feeling. Sometimes negative feelings are so deeply buried within us that it is hard to even recognize them. They often will manifest as physical symptoms, unknown fears or feelings of self-doubt, lack of self-worth, or other limitations. Look for ways to release these negative burdens. How can you take better care of yourself emotionally?

If you have regrets about any aspect of your life, do what you can to clean them up. Know that you have done the best that you knew how at the time. It's easy to look back and feel guilty or criticize your choices. Don't beat yourself up for the rest of your life. Forgiving yourself and your loved ones will bring some peace.

## Dealing with Dis-Ease

Take responsibility for the illness you are experiencing. Remember that a diagnosis is a process not an endpoint. A diagnosis is not a death sentence; it is a wake-up call and an opportunity to find a better way to care for yourself. The most important thing for anyone dealing with disease is to honor and appreciate where you are and to get the most out of life. Don't give up. Let go of drama and the things that don't support you. Love with all your heart. Do more of the things that you're passionate about, because that has tremendous healing power. Own it. Assess the benefits and the lesson behind the dis-ease. If you can't figure them out, then ask. Pray. Seek. Open and call in to you the answers that you need. Spend time in self-reflection. There is a pearl of wisdom if you take time to notice. Sit down and ask yourself these questions:

- *When did this begin?*
- *What were the first signs or symptoms that I*

*experienced?*

- *When did I become suspicious and begin to question what was happening?*
- *What was the first onset of symptoms?*
- *What were my first thought patterns about it?*
- *What did I believe?*
- *Why may I have gotten this?*
- *Which of my actions may have contributed?*
- *What benefits do I get from it?*
- *Who pays more attention to me now?*
- *What needs does this fill?*
- *Where do I not feel safe?*
- *What are the barriers to this healing?*
- *How may I get the answers I need?*
- *Who can I reach out to for help?*
- *What do I need to heal? Perhaps it is direction, guidance, a miracle.*
- *What are the lessons I am learning?*
- *How determined am I to heal this?*
- *What would it mean to me if I were free of these symptoms?*
- *What tools can I implement?*
- *Am I willing to consider visualization?*
- *Can I forgive other people who may have contributed in some way?*
- *Can I forgive myself for my actions and choices?*
- *Am I willing to consider some form of affirmations?*

If you need help, find a practitioner who listens to you that you trust. There is no consistency among practitioners, so it is difficult to compare them to one another. Everyone has different levels of expertise and uses different modalities. Embrace this, and find one you like and one that is truly working to help you. You should have the sense that your practitioner(s) and medical team are partners in your health.

Remove the barriers and be ready for change. Welcome healing. Learn to say “no” when something doesn’t serve you or others in a way that is in alignment with who you are. Say “no more” to one thing you are doing that does not serve you, that you do not want to be doing, or that you are just doing to please someone else. You should identify these things and release them from your life. Take an inventory of the people who suck the life out of you, the habits you have that are not contributing to your well-being, the things you do that waste your time, the parts of your job or business that you always put off because you don’t like dealing with them, the things that you do that you might dread or even simply feel indifferent about. Simply saying “no more” to those things makes room in your life for something better. It is difficult to make changes at first. Do one small thing at a time. You will find it is easier to adapt once you decide to stop doing something that doesn’t serve you and you take even the smallest action toward a more vibrant, healthy lifestyle.

We can't always fight the bad. Sometimes we must resolve ourselves to nurture the good. That is the crux of self-help. Contemplate what the gifts are that come from this state of dis-ease. What lessons are you learning from it? What is the biggest takeaway? What are you doing to nurture yourself? For those who have survived a major medical crisis, one of the most profound things you can do is release your fear of going through it again. Continue with healthy lifestyle changes and self-care practices. Visualize your body as healthy and vibrant.

Taking responsibility gives you great power. Seek the truth. Share your story so you can inspire others. Know that not everyone will believe you or want to hear what you have to say. This is okay because everyone is not ready to receive the information. I share my knowledge whenever I can, but I do not force it on anyone. It saddens me because I know I can help many more people than I do. It breaks my heart that many people are not open to exploring their options or trusting better ways because they have been so programmed to believe there is only one right way.

Many people are caring for a child, an elderly parent, or a family member with special needs. If this is you, take good care of your physical and emotional needs too. It is easy to neglect yourself while you are caring for someone else. You cannot effectively help your loved one if you are exhausted and run-down. An airline will tell you to put your own mask on before assisting any other passengers because you cannot benefit anyone else if you run out of oxygen. Remember, self-care is most important at times when life requires us to take care of others.

## Self-Care and Balance

Mahatma Gandhi said, "Freedom isn't worth having if it doesn't include the freedom to make mistakes." We have all neglected ourselves, abused our bodies, or made mistakes with our health. It is time to make a shift to self-care. Self-care starts with recognizing where we have failed, accepting ourselves as we are today, taking responsibility, and making a commitment to ourselves. Forgive yourself, your life, the system, God, and others for any difficult experiences you have had so you will no longer feel victimized.

Our level of empowerment is in direct proportion to our level of commitment to it. If we resign ourselves to a negative outcome, that is likely what we will experience. If we expect a better outcome and are determined to experience it, it is more likely that is what we will get.

The most important thing you can do for yourself is prioritize your own care. Self-care is not selfish. I contributed a chapter to a book about cancer. A deck of inspirational cards was developed with a quote from each author which summed up their message or stood out with great importance. These decks were given out at a fundraiser for the Teddy Bear Cancer Foundation. The quote they pulled from my chapter simply read, "Self-care is not selfish." It struck me because it is a message that I often need most. Even though I wrote that line, and I believe it to be essential to good health, I find myself struggling to practice adequate self-care. I have found that this is a critical step to good health. Most of us need more self-care. Without it, it is difficult to heal. To establish self-care, find and incorporate the perfect balance of sleep, healthy fuel, and joy into your daily routine.

### *Sleep*

Sleep is crucial to not only give your body time to rest, but also to heal, rebuild, and restore. We don't all require eight hours of sleep per night. Some of us require more. Some of us require less. Some of us need naps. Evaluate your sleep patterns and ensure that you are getting the appropriate amount of sleep. You should be waking up feeling well rested. If you are not getting enough sleep, find out why. Set boundaries. Listen to your body. If you need to rest or have time to yourself, take the time you need. You may be able to fix the problem simply by making behavioral changes, such as reducing anxiety or turning off lights or electronics a specific length of time prior to going to bed.

You may need to distance yourself from sources of Wi-Fi devices, radiofrequency, or electromagnetic radiation. You may need to make nutritional changes, such as cutting out caffeine or not eating for a specific number of hours prior to going to bed. Furthermore, you may benefit from adding supplements to correct hormonal imbalances or nutritional deficiencies, or you may need to seek medical assistance to evaluate a more serious problem.

### *Healthy Fuel*

Nurturing your body can take many forms. Make positive lifestyle changes so you can improve your health. Eliminate any food you are sensitive to. This food will weaken your energy and your body. Eat a variety of organic produce. Focus on the process of recovering, healing, and nurturing your body to optimal health.

What are possible sources of toxicity in your body? Review Chapter 4 on "The Hidden Toxins on Your Table." There is a place deep within you that knows and will recognize the truth. It is not clouded by judgment, logic, or ego.

Adopt healthy eating habits. Remember your diet either fuels your body or causes harm. Make healthy food choices as often as possible. There will be times when you have less control over what you are eating, as is the case when someone else is preparing your food. Feeling guilty while eating is not a pleasant experience. Do the best you can, enjoy yourself, and get back on track as soon as possible.

Fuel yourself with food and beverages that make you feel good and give you energy. Eat food in its most natural state. Take time to enjoy the food you are eating. Chew it thoroughly; notice the textures and flavors. Enjoy the experience.

### *Make Time for Joy*

Carve a half hour out of your schedule. You may find that you can easily reduce the amount of time you spend watching television, on social media, playing computer games, or doing things that do not add value to your life. Spend some time outside each day. Spend some time each day disconnected from all of your electronics. Enjoy time in nature. Fresh air, sunshine, and being alone to experience the quiet and solitude in your life have tremendous healing power. Make time for spiritual practice or doing things that bring you peace.

Make a commitment to get your body moving. If you do not currently have an exercise routine, begin one now. Even if it is simply to spend that extra half hour walking around the block and stretching. If you can incorporate yoga, Pilates, cardio, or weight bearing exercises, you will benefit on many levels.

Consider alternative therapies that make you feel uplifted and more balanced. Perhaps you would benefit from a massage, acupuncture, sound healing, meditation, aromatherapy, or GetSet Tapping. Remember to take time for fun, whatever that looks like to you, even if it is simply to stay home and watch a funny movie.

Part of self-care involves doing things that bring you joy. Think about what gives you a sense of passion and purpose. If you could have anything you wanted and be all that you were meant to be, what would that look like to you?

I come to life when I share the truth. What makes you come to life? How can you contribute or give back? Is there some way that you can contribute to a cause that you care about? This is not only about our own health, but our evolution as a species. Life is conspiring for us. We are all evolving and learning to trust the process of life and to live from the heart. We are all here to help each other along the journey. Each day we are given the opportunity to become a little more of who we came into this world to be.

Self-care is one of the most important points of emphasis to support your overall health and well-being. If you do not care for yourself, you will likely experience tremendous consequences and side effects. You have only one body, one mind, and one life. Take the time and energy to create a meaningful life filled with self-love, self-respect, and self-care.

# Chapter 10

# Spiritual Practice

Medicine hasn't always been practiced as it is today. In fact, it was once extraordinarily different, with many more layers and options. Traditional medicine now leads the way, and we have transformed into a very treatment-oriented and prescriptive-based society. Sick? Take these antibiotics. Headache? How about an MRI or CT scan to see what's going on? Torn ligament? Surgery can fix that. Now, modern-day medicine has remarkable benefits, but we have completely forgotten about and left behind some of the most powerful and wonderful means of preventative treatment. Options are plenty, but we should turn back the hands of time and consider all options we have available, not just the traditional ones.

There were some very sound medical practices in ancient Egypt some 3,000 to 5,000 years ago. Healers were not singular in nature. In fact, most healers were a combination of priest, doctor, and magician. They combined spiritual, scientific, and mystical principles and practices to prevent sickness and heal ailments. They used a more holistic approach to healing, one that focuses on the whole, not just one singular medical issue. These healers believed cells in the body had physical and spiritual properties, so they responded by using prayer, rituals, herbs, and detoxification, while also mixing in the crucial foundations of medicine.

Somewhere during our medical development, we have separated these practices and left many of them behind. Some have been sensationalized and capitalized upon, and others largely discredited and lost until recently. But exciting things are occurring in the realm of healing. We are once again beginning to understand the value of integrating multiple approaches to both prevent and heal complicated medical conditions.

Implementing spiritual practices such as meditation, prayer, community, and ritual can help bring you into alignment with who you are truly meant to be. Studies have proven that those who implement spiritual practices heal faster. Meaningful experiences bring you to the highest expression of your soul and create an environment for healing. That said, this chapter will help you better understand the age-old healing and preventative medical practices that have often gone lost. Once you understand all available options, you can choose what is best for you and your body and then implement different approaches that may substantially reshape your health.

Let's consider each of these options.

## Meditation

For the first time in hundreds of years, meditation is gaining widespread popularity and support from the medical community and society as a whole. Because the mind and body are so seemingly connected, healing the mind often prevents substantial issues with your body. Meditation provides clear benefits to the immune and nervous systems. Practicing meditation boosts the immune system by increasing antibodies. It also reduces inflammation, stimulates the parasympathetic nervous system by reducing stress and increasing the feeling of well-being, increases blood flow and oxygenation, reduces blood pressure, and relieves pain. It is also an effective way to unwind, reduce the stress response, experience peace, and quiet your mind. When we become more grounded and peaceful, we can carry this peace out into the world. We all live extremely hectic and stressful lives, and meditation helps to turn down the noise and improve our overall attitude and happiness. Even better, it is free and can be done almost anywhere and at your convenience, with just a small amount of time and energy. You can increase your sense of peace and refocus your day in as little as ten or twenty minutes. Meditation also gives you a deeper level of awareness and can provide you with messages that come directly from a higher Source, simply by asking.

Now, many people feel as if meditation is "woo-woo" and have trouble recognizing its value. Once they do, they still feel overwhelmed as to how they should meditate. If you are new to meditation, I would suggest you begin with a guided meditation. It might feel a little awkward at first. You will eventually feel a sense of familiarity and ease when you meditate. You may find it hard to stay focused, and you may find your mind drifting elsewhere. Regular practice will make it easier to remain focused and accomplish your goals during this quiet time.

One of the greatest aspects of meditation is that you get to choose those topics you focus on. You get to pick your awareness each time you meditate. For instance, you can fill your heart with love. Feel it expand and open and allow the love to pour forth from you. There is an endless supply when you keep it circulating. As you begin the practice of meditation, you may also find the answers to the mysteries of life by simply asking for them. Listen for the messages that come from your soul. In the beginning, the most difficult part is to trust those messages. You may feel you are not getting any messages, or the messages you are getting do not make sense. As you get more comfortable and learn to trust them and yourself, you will soon realize that they are never wrong. You will likely find the answers are quite simple and seem profound yet obvious.

Be persistent and continue to meditate on a daily basis. If meditation is not for you, don't give up on finding a place to enjoy some quiet time by yourself. If you have trouble with a specific meditation, then find another one that you are more comfortable with. As soon as you have finished meditating, write down any messages you received in a journal. Return to those messages when you can, and contemplate what they mean. You can ask for guidance or direction. Once you feel comfortable meditating, you can begin your own meditation practice. Ask specific questions, and practice being still to hear the answers to those questions. Be open to seeing signs throughout the day that relate to those questions. It is all connected in some way. For some, their answers show up in the form of signs or images. Notice the things that jump out at you. Everything is happening around you for a reason. Ask or pray that your messages come only from God, your higher self, or a trusted Source.

Consider asking these questions while you meditate:

- *What is the best path for me right now?*
- *How can I best serve the world?*
- *Is it in my best interest to____?*
- *Who am I?*
- *Why am I here?*
- *What do I need to know?*
- *What is my next step?*
- *What am I supposed to do?*
- *What can I do to help myself with _____?*
- *What am I missing?*

It is human nature to question the messages or even to judge them once received. Our judgments come from our programming and not from our higher self. Work hard not to judge the message. This isn't always easy, but it is essential. I have changed the entire course of my life as a result of messages I received. My work, my personal life, and those causes I support all directly relate to how I have been spiritually guided. For example, in one meditation, I asked if I should write another book. Despite the fact that I have written many books, writing another one was never a part of my plan.

Through my quiet time, I received the message that I needed to write a book to help people with grief. It made sense to me because one of my jobs was in a funeral home, and I had always felt a calling to work with children. I specifically asked if I was to write a book for children or adults. The response? "Both." Tears streamed down my face as I began to question how on Earth I was going to write two more books in addition to everything else I was doing. I was running my own business and working three jobs at the same time. After a few days of resisting, I knew what I had to do. I began to take action, and these books will be a result of the guidance I received.

I know these are resources needed in the world. While I never expected to be the one to do this work, I know that it is meant for me to do. I would never have started writing this book or the grief book had it not been for the messages I received. If I had discounted them or decided I did not have the time to do it, I would have never completed it. I would have neglected part of my purpose in life and the evolution of my soul. I would also have cheated countless children out of the opportunity to experience a little more peace during their grief journey and would not have contributed to my purpose of helping people find a better way to heal their lives.

When you meditate, know that you may not necessarily like the messages you receive. You might not know how you are going to act on the message. You may not know which steps you should take next. When I received the message about my smart meter, it completely shocked me. I never would have figured it out on my own. No diagnostic test would have found this answer. The answer I received changed the course of my life. Not only did that message keep me alive, it has caused me to devote a large part of my future to educate the world on the dangers of technology. Continue to ask questions. You will never be misguided. Meditation is a beautiful opportunity to connect your mind to your body. It helps to heal the soul and gain monumental and meaningful perspective when you practice it regularly and make it a ritual.

## Ritual

Meditation is just one example of an important ritual to make part of your journey. Work hard to establish daily practices that can take the form of a ritual. Some of the most common rituals might be setting aside time for prayer, reflection, visualization, a walk, yoga, time in nature, lighting a candle, setting your intentions for the day, writing in a gratitude log, or journaling. It is a routine practice that is uplifting and gives you a sense of connecting to your highest version of yourself.

There are an endless variety of rituals available to you. They can include the celebration of Mass, prayer groups, or meditation both privately and in a group setting. It may be as simple as putting your hand on your heart and asking your Source for strength, courage, or direction. They may also include giving thanks and blessing your food or water. A ritual is a practice that has a beginning and an end. The goal is that you are present in the moment and thankful for all that life has to offer.

By putting your practices into the form of a ritual, you make them sacred. You are declaring that your spiritual growth and well-being are a priority to you and your life. I find journaling to be a particularly important part of a daily ritual. To help bring these rituals to life, keep pen and paper handy, writing down pertinent and valuable information that can help you build and generate habits. In *Outside In*, a book I am coauthoring with my three sons, we provide inspiration to guide you through the journaling process that we believe is key to discovering your purpose and living the life you want.

Rituals come in many shapes and sizes. You may experience your faith and religion as a form of ritual. For example, many people make prayer part of their daily ritual. Pray for inspiration, enlightenment, and guidance. Pray for the answers that you need in order to live the life you are meant to lead. Pray with gratitude for your life and all that is a part of it. Pray for others. Pray or set the intention that you will be used for the highest good of all. There are so many reasons to pray.

Rituals eventually become habits, and you are capable of steadily relying on these habits to help you create a successful and meaningful life. So take the time to meditate, find your balance and harmony, and then implement rituals into your life.

## Community and Connection

There was a time when medicine was extremely dependent on community and connection. Historically, people worked together as a tribe, they hunted and gathered, they constructed and created, and families stayed together. As people became more independent and technology improved, many of these connections deteriorated. To that end, families and small villages would also come together and collaborate to pray for healing of their loved ones. They would work to help each other. Times have changed, and we are not as readily dependent on community and connection for healing. We go to our local doctor and rely on the advice and guidance he or she offers. We rarely seek second opinions and do not turn to our friends, neighbors, and loved ones for healing. Sickness is often done in solidarity.

It is easy to live in near solitude. We are at a point in time where you no longer need to talk to your families, spend the day interacting with coworkers, bring your check to the bank and speak to the teller, talk to a cashier at the grocery store, or sit down at a restaurant for a meal. The conveniences of modern life have created conditions where people never need to leave their house, meet their neighbors, or experience anything outside of the walls of their home. We can work remotely, do all of our financial business online, order food, groceries, meals, and goods to be delivered to our house, and do most of our correspondence electronically. You could experience all of your entertainment on your computer or in front of your television. These conveniences are making us lose a sense of community.

It is no longer necessary to interact with others. While this may be quicker and seem easier to some, at a deeper level, we crave the connections we have lost. We all want meaningful interactions with people we enjoy being around, with whom we are comfortable being our true selves.

Social media is giving people a sense of community that has largely gone missing in modern life. Almost instantly after we post something, we may have ten or twenty or possibly hundreds of people responding that they care about what we share. It feels almost as comforting as your grandma's chicken soup, and it is becoming the norm. But the truth is that this sense of existence is frail and simply cannot compare with what we gain by connecting in person with our loved ones.

We all get busy with our lives and many of us drift apart from people we once spent a lot of time with. While interacting electronically provides a sense of community, it is not enough. It does not give us the same level of satisfaction as interacting in person. At a core level, we are lonely amidst all of the incoming messages and notifications. We need to look someone in the eye, to share a hug, and to see facial expressions and hear intonations in someone's voice. There is no substitute for that physical presence.

Reconnect with friends or family in person. Take the initiative to set up a meeting. Set up a family potluck meal, make a coffee date with an old friend, or plan a lunch or dinner date. Allow time to catch up, and put your phones away. Be fully present. True connections with people you have lost contact with often withstand the test of time. They help you heal, improve your health, support the ones you love, and offer you the emotional support you need. We need to have a sense of connection and of belonging. It is great to have friends and family members to spend time and share experiences with. Not every one of those relationships provides us with the level of connection we desire. Some of us would benefit from a deep level of connection outside of our normal circle of family and friends.

Find a group of likeminded people that you can connect with who are looking to connect with people just like you. If you can't find one, start one. I belong to several groups that meet in a structured way. We share common interests, are positive, supportive, and respect each other exactly where we are. We can be vulnerable and truthful about who we are, where we are, what we need, and we keep each other on track to do what we are here to do. We have strict ground rules about showing up, being in integrity, and keeping each other accountable. At some level, each of us craves this type of connection, and sadly, most of us don't have it. Once you have a circle of friends like this, where you won't be judged or criticized, you are free to express and discover who you truly are and why you are meant to be here. You might wonder how this helps your overall health. The truth is that the notion of wellness is a cohesive one, with a balance of the body and the mind. You cannot heal one without the other. We are supplementing traditional Western medicine with a more holistic and whole body approach.

Use connection to your benefit. Take time to connect with the Earth. Spend time in nature. Spend time in silence. Appreciate the magnificence of all things. Watch the sunset. Spend time near water even if it is a small pond. Watch a spider spin its web. Walk barefoot on the wet grass. Play with a puppy. Feel the warmth of the sun on your face. Study a leaf. Hold a baby. Watch a fish swim. Listen to a bird sing. Experience nature in all its splendor. Most importantly, use community and the world around you to connect to life and create balance and harmony within your heart and soul.

## Find Meaning in Life

We each have a responsibility to determine what brings us meaning. It can be anything that makes your heart sing, makes you feel alive, and makes you feel fully engaged. Meaning equates to purpose, and purpose keeps us motivated and alive. Meaningful experiences can foster an environment for healing in our bodies. To do that, reflect on what brings you meaning and work on incorporating more meaningful experiences into your life. It may help to ask yourself the following questions:

- *What makes me feel alive?*
- *If I could do anything with my day, what would I choose?*
- *What do I love doing? What excites me?*
- *What are the best memories of my life? What did I experience in those moments?*
- *What qualities are most important to me?*
- *Which activities give me a sense of purpose?*
- *Who would I most love to serve?*
- *If I weren't afraid, what would I do?*
- *What would I do if no one were watching or if others wouldn't judge me?*
- *Are there steps I can take to be more authentic and honor my true self?*
- *What are my natural gifts or talents? What am I good at?*
- *How can I shine my light more brightly in the world?*
- *If I could do one thing with my life, what would I love to do?*

- *Where have I been wounded, and what skills has the experience given me?*
- *How can I best serve humanity by stepping into who I truly am?*
- *What would I like to accomplish?*
- *How will I feel when I accomplish this?*

These are important questions to consider when determining your true passion and purpose. After answering these questions, you may have a clearer idea of what brings you meaning. Think about the small steps you can take to ensure you are adding more meaningful experiences to your life on a daily basis. Can you incorporate more meaning into your job or business? Are there things you need to stop doing to make room in your life for more meaning? Be mindful that it is all about the journey. Don't get so caught up in the end result that you lose sight of the present moment.

Each of the sections in this chapter should help you maintain a healthy lifestyle focused on wellness and the entire picture. We often care only for one piece of the puzzle, and it comes at the expense of others. Think of that CEO who works tirelessly to provide his family financial security but doesn't go to the gym or eat right. He is serving his family at a high level but won't be around to recognize the success. We live in a modern era with remarkable medical procedures and treatment, but wouldn't it be even better if you prevented the need for these treatments in the first place?

Focus your energy on the body and the mind, realizing that you can supplement traditional medicine with a more rounded approach that is preventative, not just reactive. Meditating, praying, creating rituals, and connecting with your community will all position you to build a life filled with wellness, meaning, and abundant health.

# Section III

# The Bridge on the Path to Wellness

The "bridge" is a place of empowerment. It is where miracles occur. You step on the bridge when you decide there is another way of life and you commit to explore your options. Our goal is to find the path that feels right for you. It involves understanding both sides of the spectrum and integrating the best each has to offer.

If you want to live your healthiest life, there are some things to consider to protect yourself from harm. The information presented in this book is not meant to scare you or confuse you. It is meant to empower you and help you find the answers that are right for you. You can attract the healing that will change the course of your life by inspiring and calling in what you need.

You must take action and implement some practical steps to be proactive about your health. Which steps can you take to improve your health and well-being? Are there patterns you can integrate to improve your quality of life? Are there behaviors you can let go of that no longer serve your best interest? Are there practices you can implement that will honor your body, mind, and soul? Are there activities you can engage in that will increase your level of joy and fulfillment? What can you do to experience more purpose and creativity? What makes you feel passionate? Your return on investment increases with each step you take on this bridge.

# Chapter 11

## Finding Another Way

The best assurance of living a healthy life is being open to integration and implementing some of the actions proposed in this book. Understanding the healing process is one of the keys to being healthy. There may not be anything wrong with your health at this time. You want to keep it that way. Whether you have a health problem or not, you have many opportunities to be proactive about your health.

Many people experience mysterious symptoms and illnesses that traditional medicine can't figure out. Some have sought treatment for years or even decades without a definitive diagnosis or significant improvement. Many continue on the same path seeking answers from the same system. They hope that medical research will figure out what is wrong with them. However, medical research does not always have the answers. It does not understand the root causes of many conditions. At some point, we either resign ourselves to continue on that same path that may never yield an answer or we decide to seek a different path.

You have tremendous power when you decide there has to be another way and determine what makes the most sense for you. When you come into alignment with that decision and call in what will work for you, the options and miracles will show up in your life. This is about considering the topics presented in this book to determine the best path for you. You wouldn't be reading this book if you didn't have a higher expectation for yourself and the motivation to live a vibrant life.

Traditional medicine is extremely adept in acute care. It is brilliant at determining the current state and following a protocol that will alleviate your symptoms, put you back together, or intervene to stop a problem in your body. Alternative medicine is a little more proactive and looks for the cause of your problems and at what needs to be done to get you well and living a more balanced life.

If you are ill, I recommend you seek medical treatment or advice from a medical professional in addition to addressing all emotional and energetic imbalances that might be occurring within your life. Eastern medicine has understood the impact of energy, emotions, and spirituality on health for thousands of years. Disease or "dis-ease" is a disruption in the energy system caused by emotional upsets, deficiencies, or toxins. While doctors practicing Western medicine have the highest intention for your healing, they often do not adequately address your emotional, energetic, and spiritual well-being. They do not look for sources of toxicity in your diet or environment. At times, they do not have safe, effective methods for dealing with emotional upsets, anxiety, and stress. Most cultures widely accept that stress is at the root of disease. We have to consider the impact of these factors on current conditions.

One of my goals is to help each side become a little more comfortable with the other. After all, isn't it all about healing? As we each heal physically and spiritually, we contribute to the well-being of the planet. There is a saying that a rising tide lifts all boats. The only way we will heal individually and as a society is if we are open to integration. To do this we must let go of our fears and judgments. We can then open ourselves to the possibilities of finding the best way for us to be healthy. Simply by considering the possibility that there could be another way gives you tremendous power to shift your body and mind into healing mode.

## Finding My Way

As discussed previously in this book, my health challenges included lupus, liver tumors, GERD, ulcers, and trigeminal neuralgia. I have experienced the devastating effects of radiofrequency electrosensitivity or EHS. People often ask me how I overcame these or how I manage them. I believe it is due to my saying "no" to the disease or condition and my commitment to finding another way.

Because I believed something would show up, it did. I did not know what it would be or how I would know what to do, but I did. I learned to surrender and trust the process of life.

Things began to come to me because of my alignment.

Inspiration, circumstances, and people seemed to show up at precisely the moment that I needed them. Looking back over the series of events, it is surreal to reminisce over the synchronicities. I had to open my mind and my heart to listen for answers. At the time I was diagnosed with these ailments, I had never heard of electro-acupuncture, or of the herbs or homeopathics that I eventually used. I had never meditated or listened for answers from a higher Source. Something inside of me knew that there had to be a better way. I completely accepted it as true, and because my actions came into alignment with that truth and the possibilities that existed, I started attracting the modalities that would work for me.

While I did seek help from the medical field in the form of diagnostic testing and, in some cases, pharmaceutical drugs, I did not use medical treatments to heal from any of the conditions I faced. I did not want to manage the problems indefinitely if there was a possibility to actually heal them. Not until I explored other options did I find what I needed to heal. The path I took was the right path for me. Medical treatment may be the right path for you. This is about inspiring you to evaluate your options and being open to finding the answers that are best for you.

## By Chance or By Choice

The current medical model often supports treating symptoms with drugs instead of finding the cause of the problem. The evolution of healing has been manipulated by a system that has monetized medicine for its benefit, not that of the patient. If you aren't experiencing the results you want, you must take responsibility for that. If there is something about your health that you don't like, you must make changes. You can heal by chance or by choice. This is about taking back your power. There is tremendous power in realizing that you have options even when you are not sure what those options are.

If anything is wrong, it is a result of our choices. It is all a result of what we feed our bodies, minds, and spirits, consciously or unconsciously, or what we are not giving them that they need, or what we are exposing them to that they do not want. There are no flaws in the physiological properties of the body. The body is much more intelligent than we will ever be. God doesn't make mistakes.

Your job is to find the best way for YOU to heal. While I am sharing my stories, I want to be perfectly clear that this is about you and giving you a different perspective and some opportunities to find a better way for you. Perhaps something I wrote in this book will call out to you and make more sense than anything else. Trust that. I encourage you to further explore and experiment with what I have said. Make some changes to your diet, lifestyle, or mindset.

Once we change our thinking, we can attract the answers or the modality that will change the course of our lives. It is that simple. What then calls to you may be the traditional route, or it may be something less conventional. Either way, it is important that you sit in that truth that there is another way. Listen for what calls to you and what your gut tells you. This is a missing link in healing. We are conditioned to go with what we know and not to question it.

A number of clients have told me that they prayed for an answer for their healing, and within a few days, someone mysteriously shared a story and gave them my business card. At a health exposition, three people came to my booth and told me they had prayed for someone to help them and somehow they knew I would be the one. One woman came up to me with tears in her eyes and asked if she could hug me. I had no idea who she was, but she explained her predicament and she believed that I would help her. She became a client who received the miracle of healing that she was seeking. These people were open to being directed to the answers they needed. Through my years of education in toxicity, deficiency, and the numerous modalities I have studied, there is often some source of advice I can offer. Ultimately it is up to the individual to decide what is best for them. While I would gladly give my opinion, I would not direct someone on the course of action to take.

The truth is that medical doctors are not educated in many or any other healing modalities. They are not trained to recognize most nutritional deficiencies or how nutrients can improve health. Dieticians do not always know what you are eating. The food they recommend is not necessarily good for you. Many dieticians or nutritionists still follow the food pyramid. They often recommend GMO food or food that contains exceptionally high levels of pesticides or preservatives. Some are not educated on the toxic properties of many food ingredients and believe that if it has been approved by a regulatory agency, then it is safe for you to consume. They mean well, but they can only teach what they have been taught academically or through their life experiences.

Good nutrition is critical to good health. Food was medicine before modern medications and the drug-oriented bias became the norm. Hippocrates said, "Let thy food be thy medicine, and thy medicine, thy food." Revelations 22:2 says that the leaves of the trees are for the healing of the nations. Many references in the Bible talk about herbs and oils such as olive leaves, frankincense, and myrrh. Somehow over the generations, the healing properties of food, herbs, and other medicinal plants have been largely ignored. Because of this, you may need to turn to other practitioners outside of the field of medicine when looking for natural remedies.

Don't leave your healing entirely up to your medical team. Each has their own specialty. For example, an oncologist is an expert and has studied cancer, how it acts in the body, which chemotherapeutants will kill it, and how to remove it. They don't know how it will work for you. They can only give you a range of possibilities and their educated guess. There are no guarantees with medicine or with any other modalities. Earlier in this book, we talked about the impact of a diagnosis, the power of belief, and the nocebo effect. If you are given a bleak prognosis, it does not mean you cannot restore your body back to perfect health. I know you can do it because I have done it.

I believe we need an integrative approach. That does not mean that traditional medicine is not part of the plan. Don't put all your eggs in one basket until you have explored all options and feel you have addressed all levels of healing that you are comfortable with. Don't only look at "reality." Look at all possibilities. If you believe it is not possible to heal, you probably won't heal. Think about what is possible for you if you were to take doubt out of the equation. Do what you can to clear out your doubts, limiting beliefs, and reservations. We are limited only by our minds, beliefs, and conditioning.

We need emotional and spiritual well-being, energetic balance, the belief that healing is possible, and the faith that we are already healing in order for healing to occur. You don't have to believe in energetic balance, but you can pray for it. You can pray that you will be restored to balance or for the understanding required for it to make sense to you. Seek an experienced practitioner or coach to help you. Realize that you do have options. My way may not be your way. Using modern medicine exclusively may be the right path for you. My intention is not to persuade you to use one type of treatment but to open your eyes, mind, and heart to other options and find the best protocol for you.

Good insurance does not ensure good health. There are no guarantees that any treatment, conventional or holistic, will work for anyone. Most medical insurance companies only cover allopathic medicine. This is a huge limiting factor for many people because holistic or alternative treatments often must be paid for out of pocket. Weigh all your options. Many of the suggestions I offer can be done on your own with minimal cost.

That point where you start to ask questions and come to believe that there has to be a better way is a tremendous moment of power. "There's got to be another way" is one of the most powerful things you can say to yourself when you don't like your options. Whether you see a medical doctor, licensed practitioner, mystic, or healer, look at the overall picture. Most of these people are extremely competent and have devoted their lives to helping people. They may have gone to medical school or followed their own path to study and find their own answers. Each has a special gift and has answered a calling. If they have unconventional views or a protocol that is not validated by medical research, it doesn't make them bad, better, or worse than anyone else. Any of the above may have a limited knowledge based on their training, education, beliefs, experiences, and gifts. The same event or illness doesn't get the same result with a single method of treatment. Two people with the same form of cancer often respond very differently to the same treatment. An allergic reaction may look the same in two people, but the culprit can be entirely different.

Traditional medicine looks at signs, symptoms, and test results that can be explained as a result of studies conducted by companies or organizations with special interests in the treatment protocol. They have largely lost sight of the truth that healing must address all contributing factors of illness including sensitivities, physical toxins, deficiencies, thought patterns, emotions, and beliefs. Medicine is evolving. They don't have all the answers. Forgive them. They are doing the best they can. It may take many years before medicine embraces an integrative approach. Right now it is up to you to make the choices that support your health and well-being.

It is not only necessary to know about all of this. You should also act upon this knowledge. Make a conscious effort to implement these steps and take action continuously toward your end goal of healing or perfect health. Healing is as much an art as it is a science. It is very spiritual in nature. There are many documented cases of healing that have defied medical explanation. I hope that you will realize you have tremendous influence over your healing. It is by choice.

## The Fall and Recognizing the Gift

Early on the morning of April 10, 2015, I took an express trip down a flight of stairs in my home. My foot slipped off the top step, and I awoke at the bottom of a steep flight of eleven steps in excruciating pain. I had dislocated my right shoulder, and the ball and socket joint was protruding out under my arm. I could not move any part of my body. The pain was unbearable. I lay at the foot of the stairs for about two hours. I knew I might remain there for three days before my son would return home from a weekend road trip. I could not get to a phone. Initially, I thought I had broken my neck. I struggled to get my thoughts together. My options were limited.

I feared that I would die there if I had broken my neck and I moved in such a way to injure my spinal cord. The thought of being permanently paralyzed circled my mind. My only options were to lie there until someone found me or to figure out a way to get myself out of this contortion predicament. I knew I had to put my fears aside if I was going to be able to take any proactive steps. As painful as it was to move, the more I thought about staying there for three days, the less I liked the idea. I began to focus all my efforts on moving my fingers. Success. Then my efforts went to my toes. I could not tell if they were moving, but I could feel the muscles in my calves moving. Good enough. With my hands and feet working, I could get somewhere.

I mustered all my strength to fight through the pain. When I realized that my arm was going backward and I would never get myself up on all fours, I decided to relocate my shoulder. I had never relocated any bone or joint before, so I wasn't sure what to do. At that point, some sort of survival instinct kicked in. I grunted and groaned as I reached over my torso with my left arm and pulled my rib cage back to center, repositioned my shoulder joint, then reached over my head and with all my might, pulled my right arm down to my side. In that moment, I realized that I had made a very important decision: I was not going to give up. I would do whatever I had to do to get myself out of that predicament. I could now move, and that was all that mattered.

I believe in noninvasive practices whenever possible. Looking back over the experience, that fateful morning taught me many important lessons. I learned a lot from the decisions I made those first few hours. In the days that followed, I chose not to undergo diagnostic testing in an effort to avoid radiation exposure. I know nothing can be done for broken ribs and shoulder blades, so I felt there was no need to be irradiated.

I eventually underwent diagnostic testing because I began to question myself and allowed fear to creep in. The testing process involved X-rays, CT scans, and an MRI. The results were pretty inconclusive, stating "no obvious spine fractures," a broken posterior rib, and six tears of the rotator cuff.

I opted not to have rotator cuff surgery. Half the doctors supported this decision. It has taken almost two years for me to heal from that fall. If I had chosen surgery, there is no way to know if I would be any better or if I would have healed any faster. There is also the possibility that I could have been worse off after the surgery. Many people get infections or have less range of motion after similar surgeries. Some need additional surgeries, multiplying the risk of problems and increasing the amount of drugs necessary. Some people suffer long-term consequences from the anesthesia. A small percentage of people have complications and die in routine surgeries. I wasn't willing to take the risk. You may be better off not seeking an invasive procedure if you are not convinced that you need it. Weigh your options. After considering mine, this was the best choice for me.

This experience gave me the gift of time. It offered me a lot of down time because I couldn't do anything that required lifting or moving that arm. I was able to contemplate and realize that I had more books to write. At the time, I was working four part-time jobs and I really had no time for anything. One of the lessons I learned was the importance of self-care. I had never learned this lesson because my life was in service to others. It was always busy and somewhat chaotic. The recovery period allowed me to contemplate what was most important in my life and put me on a different path.

Initiation is the journey by which you discover more about yourself and gain peace and a deeper understanding of life. You can consciously choose this journey or you can be forced through it by experiences or the traumas of everyday life. You often don't see the lessons while you are in the midst of the experience. It is not until later that you can look back and see it from a different, more evolved perspective.

Illness or injury is a wake-up call and provides an opportunity to explore and to learn more about your true self and your purpose and passions. Always look for the gift and lesson behind the symptom, illness, or problem. No matter what the setback, find the gift.

### Where to Start and How to Find Your Way

If you are facing a health challenge, start by asking your doctor for another option. Your doctor will often give you options if he or she is open to helping you find the treatment plan that is best for you. In some cases, your doctor may feel your condition is too serious to risk avoiding a specific treatment. I have witnessed doctors give patients the option of some time to remedy a problem with diet, exercise, supplements, or holistic practices. I have also witnessed these same doctors tell patients their condition is too serious and advise them to start a traditional treatment immediately. If waiting to start a treatment poses a threat to your health, respect their opinion. If the doctor is simply not willing to consider any other way, I recommend finding another doctor.

It is not important that you do all the research and figure

it out for yourself. It is necessary that you acknowledge that there is another way. You don't have to know the way. The future of healing lies in our ability to realize how unique we are. We must follow our own path. We have a tendency to put ourselves in boxes. Explore the possibility of how it might feel to step outside of the box.

God did not create us to be victims, to be unconscious, or to be mediocre. He created us to be magnificent expressions of ourselves. Everyone can rise above his or her limits and programming. Whenever we are faced with adversity, whether it is in heath or any other area of life, we have the freedom to choose which action to take.

James Allen said, "A man's mind may be likened to a garden, which may be intelligently cultivated or allowed to run wild; but whether cultivated or neglected, it must, and will, bring forth." Make choices that will bring about the result you want. When you don't take action to change something, you are choosing to let it remain the same.

Be aware that you will experience conflict when you are attached to a different outcome. Pay attention to what your feelings are telling you. Know that you can shift your focus onto a new outcome. Be willing to experience something different. You can then choose to boldly step onto a new path that will put you in the direction that you want to go.

If you are healthy, ask yourself if there are changes you can make to ensure you stay healthy. If you are experiencing a symptom, have been given a diagnosis, or put on a treatment, and you are looking for another way or a different reality, there are things you can do to decide if there is a better way or a different path for you. Consider these possibilities:

- *Ask your doctor about any risks and benefits of any treatment or procedure.*
- *Ask your doctor for another option.*
- *If you are not satisfied, find another doctor or get a second opinion.*
- *Set aside any judgments of medical principles and alternative techniques.*
- *Consider a doctor who practices functional medicine or is open to integrative medicine.*
- *Find a holistic practitioner. Ask for a recommendation from friends, family, co-workers, or a local health food store if you don't know someone.*
- *Pay close attention to what your body is telling you.*
- *Log any symptoms or observations you feel might be related.*
- *Log everything you ingest or apply to your body to see if there is a correlation.*
- *Consider having a sensitivity screening to see if there are products or food that cause your body a negative response. In my experience, it is much more helpful than allergy tests.*
- *Take a toxin inventory and make any changes to your*

*lifestyle to reduce your exposure.*

- *Ask yourself if anything you read in this book jumped out at you.*
- *Ask or pray for the answers to come to you and that you will notice them.*
- *Sit in meditation and listen for answers. Listen to the whispers from your soul.*
- *Visualize and feel yourself free from the problem.*
- *Write an affirmation in gratitude for the outcome you expect.*
- *Pay attention to the answers that show up.*
- *If you need help, pray that God or the universe puts the perfect physicians, specialists, modalities, and practitioners in your path and for the capacity to recognize them.*
- *Honor your feelings.*
- *Follow your gut instincts.*
- *Be willing to experience something different.*
- *Remember that when you are in alignment with a specific outcome, life will take care of the details. You don't have to figure it all out on your own.*

Life is always conspiring for you. Trust the process of life. There is a reason you hold this book in your hands right now. If you have no idea where to start to better your health, go somewhere you can be out of the distractions of everyday life. Turn off the television or radio, turn off your phone, and go to a quiet area outside or within your home, even if it has to be the bathroom. Take a few deep breaths and get centered. Look at your feet on the floor. Close this book. Close your eyes and say a prayer or ask your inner wisdom for answers. Ask for what you need to know to remedy your current situation. You can even ritualize this process. Ask to be divinely guided. Treat it as a sacred experience to access a higher source of wisdom. Then open this book to a random page. I believe so strongly that the universe gives us exactly what we need in any given moment that I will say the page you open this book to is not random at all. You opened to it because there is something on it that you need to consider. Read over the page until something jumps out at you. I am not suggesting the answer to every problem in life is answered in this book. Trust that it will trigger some piece of wisdom that will steer you in the right direction. Expect a miracle.

# Chapter 12

# Integration

The bridge is about integration. It is the metaphorical place where true wellness happens, where traditional and holistic healthcare meet, and where miracles can occur. The bridge is where science and spirituality meet. It is where medicine and nature meet. It is where mind and body meet. It involves finding balance in life and partnering with medical doctors and holistic practitioners that honor you. The magic occurs when you find that balance. It is a place where we are restored to wholeness.

Here we consider the importance of taking care of our physical bodies along with nurturing our souls, providing proper nutrients, and developing the mindset to not only elevate our health but to thrive in living a joyful, purpose-driven life. It is from this place that we can explore the opportunities our lives hold. The lessons you learn here about health can be applied to any area of your life.

Ancient Egyptian healing integrated the mind, body, and spirituality. Sadly, we have largely shut down integration as a society. We have essentially outlawed some techniques or threatened practitioners with criminal charges. In our society today, you have to be a licensed medical professional to heal someone. If you heal someone without the proper credentials, you can be imprisoned for it. If you heal after using a nonconventional method, it is often considered spontaneous healing.

Traditional medicine has a tendency to take a strong stance against holistic principles. It often criticizes and discredits anyone who thinks outside the box. It condemns "New Age" principles and labels any studies or testimonies as pseudoscience. Yet, we are finding more and more evidence of people staying healthy or becoming healthy again when they embrace an alternative practice. We are finding that going back to "age-old" principles offers resolution to many people's health challenges.

Right now, the world is in too much competition to encourage integration. Too many industries want all of the control and all of the money. We are moving toward a system of standardizing medicine for the population and focusing mainly on the bottom line. We are moving away from individualized care between a doctor and a patient.

There is a lot of judgment about one form of healthcare over the other. Judgment is often fueled by fear. Clarity dissipates fear. It is human nature for anyone who has been strongly conditioned to believe that everything they have been taught is "truth" to then have a hard time opening up to other beliefs. Ideally, each side should agree to honor and respect the other. We are working hard as a society to forgive the wounds we have created in the past: segregation and discrimination, chaos, and violence. Yet we continue to suffer needlessly in the area of healthcare because of this disconnect. We all need to love, accept, and respect each other simply because we have each come into the world to fulfill a purpose.

We are learning that we must look beyond the physical body. We are becoming more willing to seek an understanding beyond traditional science. We are beginning to truly understand that addressing only one part of the body without addressing the other is not enough. Treating the body without looking at the mind is not enough. Treating a symptom or managing a disease without looking for a cause will not serve us over the long term. It will not be as effective to treat the body without incorporating self-care and spirituality.

We are living in a very exciting time. Scientific discoveries are constantly happening around us. Medicine and diagnostic equipment have become incredibly innovative. The rediscovery of the wisdom of ancient techniques and traditions is shifting our paradigms and beliefs. It is not only possible, but quite simple to tap into the greatest healing power that exists. We can live our best lives by making informed decisions and integrating the best practices from each discipline.

## What if . . .?

No one wants to get to the end of their life and realize there are a lot of things left undone. No one wants to leave this life with regrets. In the end, we want to celebrate our lives.

We want to be happy with who we are and who we became through the journey. Make the most of the time you have and do those things that are important to you and that give you a sense of joy and accomplishment.

Some people outright decide to abuse their bodies. Nowhere is the impact of abuse on the human body more obvious than in the case of some of the most famous musicians and entertainers. They had fortune and fame. Financially they were wealthy beyond most people's comprehension. Yet, they lost their lives because of the choices they made. Think about legendary musicians and entertainers such as Janis Joplin, Jim Morrison, Jerry Garcia, Jimi Hendrix, Elvis, Whitney Houston, Johnny Cash, Kurt Cobain, Ernest Hemingway, Michael Jackson, John Belushi, and Marilyn Monroe. What might these people have gone on to accomplish had they honored their bodies and minds, gotten the help they needed, and taken better care of themselves?

Everyone has a contribution to make. There have been many famous contributors to the world in the form of innovations, works of art, science, philanthropy, and entertainment. Think about how different the world would be if some of these contributors had died as a result of making uninformed or poor choices before they made their contribution.

What if Michelangelo had died from an adverse drug reaction before sculpting David, painting the Sistine Chapel, and influencing the Renaissance art period?

What if Thomas Edison had died from complications related to eating pesticide-ridden fruit before he invented the lightbulb?

What if Alexander Graham Bell had died from esophageal cancer related to eating genetically modified corn and soy before inventing the telephone in 1876?

What if Mother Teresa had died from a brain tumor from sleeping with her cell phone without ever influencing world peace?

What if Jane Goodall hadn't realized her African power company had put a smart meter on her hut, and as a result developed Alzheimer's disease before being able to study the chimpanzees and contribute to animal rights?

What if Jackie Robinson had died because he accepted a diagnosis and prognosis without ever looking for the cause or another way to heal before breaking the racial barrier in baseball?

What if Martin Luther King Jr. had died from kidney failure resulting from diabetes caused by years of drinking diet soda and eating sugary snacks before making his impact on civil rights?

What if Shakespeare had committed suicide after years of struggling with anxiety and depression caused by exposure to electromagnetic radiation without ever creating his great literary works?

What if these people had not known there were dangers lurking around the choices they were making? What if they had trusted others to look out for them? What if they had been warned about the dangers but thought it would never happen to them? What if they had believed they could live a risky lifestyle and that their doctors would later be able to fix them with a magic pill?

Luckily, the hypothetical situations presented above did not occur and each of the individuals made notable contributions to the world. They were not faced with many of the environmental challenges we face today. The good news is that we know the dangers. We know what to look out for. We know how to drive changes in the world. We have the freedom of choice to protect ourselves and to take the best possible care of ourselves and our loved ones.

When you make choices without considering the harm that could be done, there are consequences. Your health may suffer and you may be deprived of many experiences. Each of us came into this life with a limited number of days. What actions will you take so you can live a healthier, more vibrant life? What can you do to minimize harmful exposures in your diet and environment? How can you experience more joy? What can you do to live with more meaning? What could extra years of vibrant health provide you in terms of experiences, fulfilling your purpose, and contributions to family and the world? What can you do with the time that you have left? I will help you explore some of these questions in the coming sections to help you realize the benefits of making informed choices and how you can have a more meaningful experience of life.

**The Path to Wellness**

Stress, deficiencies, exposure to sensitivities, pathogens, or toxins can all cause illness. Healing comes when you give your body what it needs physically, nutritionally, emotionally, and spiritually. Health and illness are about our choices. They are not a matter of luck. Every choice you make impacts your body.

We all have the freedom of choice. When you feel that life is spinning out of control, know that you have complete control over the questions that you ask, the mindset that you have, the faith that you surrender to a higher Source, the courage you muster, the hope that you create, and the ability that you have to trust your heart and gut.

To heal, we must be willing to accept change. We may need to change our attitudes, habits, beliefs, and be willing to release ourselves from a victim mentality. When we do, we will begin to realize that things do not happen to us, they happen for us at a soul level. No matter how difficult our experiences may seem in the moment, they happen for our growth.

This is really a conversation about empowerment. You have to make the decision to be empowered. You have more power over your circumstances than you may realize.

It is up to you to decide if you will let your struggles define you in a way that holds you back indefinitely or encourages you to grow stronger and more confident.

It is possible that you might not fully heal from a given obstacle. We obviously will all transition from this world. It is all about the choices you make while you are here and the quality of the life you lead. You can live your life in dis-ease or disease, but you don't have to. It's simply whether you are truly ready to heal and transform the illness, ask the right questions, and find and stick to the plan that is for your highest good and believe it is done.

When we take away the things that negatively impact our bodies, give them the support they need, the movement they crave, and recognize what is not working, we open up to the answers and possibilities of living a vibrant life. Look at things with an open mind. Work on eliminating negative influences from your life, seeking positive influences, improving the quality of the food you eat, detoxifying your environment, and coming to peace with your emotions.

Expand your views as you go forward. Follow your heart. Trust in a higher Source. Ask questions. Explore. Know that anything is possible. Everything is curable. There is always another way. Trust your gut, believe in your inner wisdom and that the universe will provide the answers. Have faith. Make choices that honor your body. It is never too late to change your mind. Believe in miracles. Sometimes we don't see the miracles because of our programming and conditioning. We just don't believe or notice that they are happening. I see them happen every day. I have seen people who were diagnosed with terminal illness heal quickly when they decide not to believe the prognosis and work on finding the solution.

Be gentle with yourself. Have compassion for yourself and others as we evolve. Do not beat yourself up for the choices you made in the past. Do not feel shame because you did not know better. The past is behind you, and there is nothing you can do right now to change it. Feeling guilt, remorse, or resentment about it will only cause you additional harm. Forgive yourself and the system. Know the truth, but forgive those who have created the problems. It will do you no good to hold on to anger.

Anger is a normal response. There are times when I get very angry about the greed and corruption that knowingly drives disease. This anger increases my stress. While it comes up often, I have learned to let it go as quickly as it comes on. I vent. I rant sometimes and get very passionate, and I tend to get angry when I speak about it. This anger drives my passion. When I am done speaking, I let it go. If I didn't, I would be allowing the system to control me. Accept that this is the way it is for now, take that information, and take responsibility for the choices you make from this point forward. Do what you can to provoke change. Know that you support the practices wherever you spend your money. Be grateful that you have this knowledge and can act upon it.

These are the choices that you have. No one can take them away from you. Only you will decide which direction you will go and whether you will give up your hope, courage, and faith. Live your best life. Break any cycles of suffering, dis-ease, and struggle. Rewrite the story of your life.

## Be the Change

How do we live in a world where our agricultural practices are poisoning us, our planet, and our atmosphere? How do we survive if our bodies do not recognize the processed and altered food we eat? How do we advance technologically when our technology is actually harming us? How do we make choices when information and truths are being suppressed? The answer is we take back our power. We get educated. We change our behaviors and habits. We become the solution.

We are living in dynamic times. We have such power to change the world. We must undo some of our programming and beliefs and then change our mindset and our behavior. I have a quote on my wall by Mahatma Gandhi that reads, "Be the change you wish to see in the world." It starts with you. You can change anything that you do not like. We can protect our planet, our food supply, and ourselves. We can do this with the choices we make and the practices we support as consumers.

You can't have sustained health without being proactive and taking precautions in the world today. Making purposeful decisions sets you up to live in a healthy, meaningful way. As a world with a population of about seven billion people, we are spending twenty-five to thirty billion dollars annually on space programs and space exploration. As a scientist, I find it extremely interesting to see pictures from space and of other planets. Is it really necessary though?

At the same time, many countries face huge national debts and cannot provide education to all children, adequately protect against terrorism and gang violence, and provide food and proper nutrition to many starving people. How much would it cost to increase the level of peace and happiness in the world? What if we put half that money into improving life? What if we committed to making the world a better place from a perspective of peace and well-being instead of fulfilling a need to satisfy our egos to be the first to make milestones in space or create technology from space to make the world run faster and more efficiently? Of course, this is not just about space. There are billions of dollars budgeted for other programs that don't contribute to people's health or well-being. In fact, some of it goes into programs and technologies that are harming people's health.

The majority of healthcare dollars go to managing chronic diseases. Wouldn't we be better served to use more money to nurture wellness? A generation ago, we were spending more on food than we were on medical care.

Today, most of us spend more on medical care than we do on food. It may serve us to rethink where we spend our money and seriously contemplate if we would rather spend it on taking care of ourselves up front or to undo the damage down the road. Many feel we can't afford a gym membership, yoga class, or organic food, but can we afford not to take care of ourselves? A health crisis is not only a financial burden, but it also takes a physical and emotional toll on the body.

## Zest for Life

Many of us spend a lot of effort trying to fit in. We work hard to blend into the norm when it is our purpose to stand out and be ourselves. We were meant to stand out. Life has chosen us to fulfill a unique purpose. This may be a specific calling, and it can take many forms. For instance, it can be to nurture our children, create something beautiful, help others, contribute to a greater cause, or expand our perspective.

We are each given gifts and talents, and when we ignore them or don't answer the call, we find ourselves in a state of disharmony or dis-ease, losing our sense of well-being, losing our sense of purpose, and becoming ill. Our gifts do not always come beautifully packaged. Sometimes they are traits that we develop as a result of difficult life circumstances and deep wounds. When we express our gifts, we often feel a zest for life.

When you love what you are doing and feel a sense of passion for life, you raise your vibration and your body begins to function harmoniously. It is then that healing is most likely to occur. Have you ever noticed that when you are doing something you are excited about or are in a new, healthy relationship, your negative thoughts, aches, and pains seem to disappear?

## Return on Investment

You may be wondering what you get in return for making these healthy choices. You may spend a little extra time educating yourself and more money buying better quality products and food, but these will pay off in terms of improved quality of life and extra life experiences.

This is not just about extending your life for the sake of living longer. It is about living the best possible life you can while you are here. It is about being healthy and vibrant so you can have more experiences. You get more opportunities. You have more moments. You get to do more. You get to be more. The world needs more experienced, enlightened people.

Perhaps this will allow you to see your favorite football team win the Super Bowl, see your baseball team win the World Series, see your children grow up, perhaps get to meet and experience your great-grandchildren, achieve a personal goal, or make a contribution to the world. Maybe you will find and fulfill your purpose, actually do your life's work instead of just wondering about it or identifying it and feeling like you don't have the energy or that there is no time to do anything about it.

This may provide you the opportunity to retire and still have many years left to enjoy. You may be able to do more work in the world. This may or may not entail a nine-to-five job. You can still make a difference in the world. It may be contributing to world peace, helping others, or may simply be that you are present for your family, that you are there by your partner's side, are there to take your grandchildren to the park, or it may provide you the chance to travel and see the world.

### Feeding Your Body, Mind, and Soul

It will always serve you to raise your vibration by focusing on what you want, surrounding yourself with healthy people, music, media, food, practices that feed your soul, and filling your life with things that are meaningful to you. This can include the arts, cultural events, philanthropic contributions, music, festivals, cooking, movement, and dance.

Look for things that give you a sense of belonging. Consider meet-up groups and connecting with likeminded people and people with similar interests. It is great to spend time in groups you are connected to that have a broad range of interests, such as family and coworkers. Spend more time with those that share similar interests that are most meaningful to you. Make a list of the things you get the most enjoyment from, and think of people you know who seem to enjoy those same things. Come up with ways you can share those experiences.

Rumi said, "When you do things from your soul, you feel a river moving in you, a joy." Feeding your soul has a healing effect on your mind and body. Think about some ways you can feed your soul. You may want to ponder these questions:

- *What can you do to have a more soulful experience of life?*
- *What do you love to do?*
- *What brings you joy?*
- *What would you love to do more of?*
- *What is meaningful to you?*
- *What makes you curious?*
- *Is there a way you can explore those things that interest you that you may have been ignoring?*
- *What makes you feel creative?*
- *How can you cultivate your passions?*
- *How can you add more creativity to your life?*
- *How can you add more positive influences to your life?*
- *Can you think of some ways to surround yourself in beauty?*
- *What can you do to expand your awareness?*
- *Which philanthropic events or organizations can you get involved with?*

- *What can you do that will give you the sense of helping others?*
- *How can you give back?*
- *What can you do to heal your heart and soul while your body is going through the journey?*
- *How do you show up in the world?*
- *How will you serve the world? The effect you have on others is what counts.*

Don't take life too seriously. Add humor and playfulness even if you have to pretend at first. Above all, take care of yourself. Take care of your needs. Do things to spoil yourself. Make self-care a priority. Remember, self-care is not selfish.

**Get Curious and Be Creative**

Curiosity may have killed the cat, but it is essential to growth and expansion. Here are some suggestions to foster the need to express creativity in everyday life. Draw a picture, doodle, color in an adult coloring book, make fun patterns in the carpet of a room that you vacuum, make neat rows the next time you cut the grass, prepare a colorful meal, write a short story, research a topic of interest, make a craft, tackle a do-it-yourself home project, design a flower bed, rearrange your furniture, take something apart and rebuild it, make a video slideshow of your favorite pictures, create a thoughtful gift for a friend, or take a hike and look for patterns that you notice in nature. As you can see, the opportunities are abundant, and as you allow yourself to become more curious and creative, you will expand your perspective and enthusiasm. You will exercise the "muscle" that helps you think outside the box.

## Create a Bucket List

Consider creating a bucket list. It is easiest to think of things you would like to do in your lifetime that are within your means or a slight stretch. If everything on the list is well above your means or feels unattainable, you will be less likely to start checking things off the list. This is not to say you don't want to have big dreams. For this exercise, focus the list on those things you know you can do but you might just feel you don't have the time to do. Once you put activities on your list, you will be more likely to take action and experience them.

Use the space that follows to create your list. Fill it with everything you can think of that you would like to experience, accomplish, or get done. Come back to it later if you need to. Just be sure to fill your list with ninety things. It may seem exhaustive, but it will make it easier to start checking things off. Here are some suggestions for the sorts of ideas you might include on your list: Create a meal for your family; organize a family get-together for no specific reason; climb Mount Kilimanjaro; visit your favorite sports team while they are on the road or visit their stadium; run a 5k; complete a triathlon; visit a state park in your area; visit the Grand Canyon; take your kids or grandkids or parents to the zoo; attend a concert; meet a friend for lunch; plan a picnic in the park with your partner or a friend; attend a play in your community or at a local high school or college; go fishing; volunteer at an animal shelter; explore a local museum; take a fun class in something that interests you; make amends with someone; go on a nature walk; experience a new cuisine or restaurant that interests you; rescue a pet; organize your closet; complete your degree; volunteer to help out at a community event; perform a random act of kindness; repair something around your home; read a book; or do a puzzle.

***My Bucket List . . .***

1. ________________________________________
2. ________________________________________
3. ________________________________________
4. ________________________________________
5. ________________________________________
6. ________________________________________
7. ________________________________________
8. ________________________________________
9. ________________________________________
10. ________________________________________
11. ________________________________________
12. ________________________________________
13. ________________________________________
14. ________________________________________
15. ________________________________________
16. ________________________________________
17. ________________________________________
18. ________________________________________
19. ________________________________________

20. ______________________________

21. ______________________________

22. ______________________________

23. ______________________________

24. ______________________________

25. ______________________________

26. ______________________________

27. ______________________________

28. ______________________________

29. ______________________________

30. ______________________________

31. ______________________________

32. ______________________________

33. ______________________________

34. ______________________________

35. ______________________________

36. ______________________________

37. ______________________________

38. ______________________________

39. ______________________________

40. ______________________________

41. ______________________________

42. ______________________________

43. ______________________________

44. ______________________________

45. ______________________________

46. ______________________________

47. ______________________________

48. ______________________________

49. ______________________________

50. ______________________________

51. ______________________________

52. ______________________________

53. ______________________________

54. ______________________________

55. ______________________________

56. ______________________________

57. ______________________________

58. ______________________________

59. ______________________________

60. ____________________________________________

61. ____________________________________________

62. ____________________________________________

63. ____________________________________________

64. ____________________________________________

65. ____________________________________________

66. ____________________________________________

67. ____________________________________________

68. ____________________________________________

69. ____________________________________________

70. ____________________________________________

71. ____________________________________________

72. ____________________________________________

73. ____________________________________________

74. ____________________________________________

75. ____________________________________________

76. ____________________________________________

77. ____________________________________________

78. ____________________________________________

79. ____________________________________________

80. ______________________________
81. ______________________________
82. ______________________________
83. ______________________________
84. ______________________________
85. ______________________________
86. ______________________________
87. ______________________________
88. ______________________________
89. ______________________________
90. ______________________________
91. ______________________________
92. ______________________________
93. ______________________________
94. ______________________________
95. ______________________________
96. ______________________________
97. ______________________________
98. ______________________________
99. ______________________________

If you did not fill the list, come back and add to it as you think of things to include. Periodically review your list and commit to start checking things off. In the end, you will find that creating this list and then fulfilling each of your goals is an extremely powerful way to live your life it to its fullest extent.

**Live Your Best Life**

Your health and happiness matter most in this world. I hope this book will help you make choices that are in alignment with your highest good. This involves making decisions about all the options you have to stay healthy and, if necessary, to reverse any damage by finding and eliminating the cause of any problems. Whenever you are not satisfied with your circumstances, know that there is always another way.

Your body is uniquely programmed to heal itself when it has what it needs and is properly cared for. You have the ability to call in the answers and resources that will work for you.

Go back and read parts of this book again slowly. There is wisdom in each idea. Not everything will resonate with you. Some ideas may seem radical. Take only those things that make sense to you and implement small changes. Each step you take is a step closer to health. Consider the possibility that this book can help you become empowered and develop a deeper understanding of healing and find the path that is right for you. Believe in the possibilities. Step boldly onto the bridge, and welcome miracles into your life.

## Final Note

The truth is you are a gift to the planet. It may be difficult for you to admit and accept your magnificence. You have influenced the world more than you will ever know. The world will never be the same because of you. You don't have to win a Nobel Peace Prize, balance the federal budget, make a scientific discovery, or solve world hunger. You just have to be you. If I could leave you with one piece of wisdom, it would be for you to know how amazing you are. You have incredible power to shape the course of your life and to welcome miracles every day. If you take nothing more than that from this book, it will have served its purpose.

May you continue to brightly shine the light of who you are in the world.

Namaste.

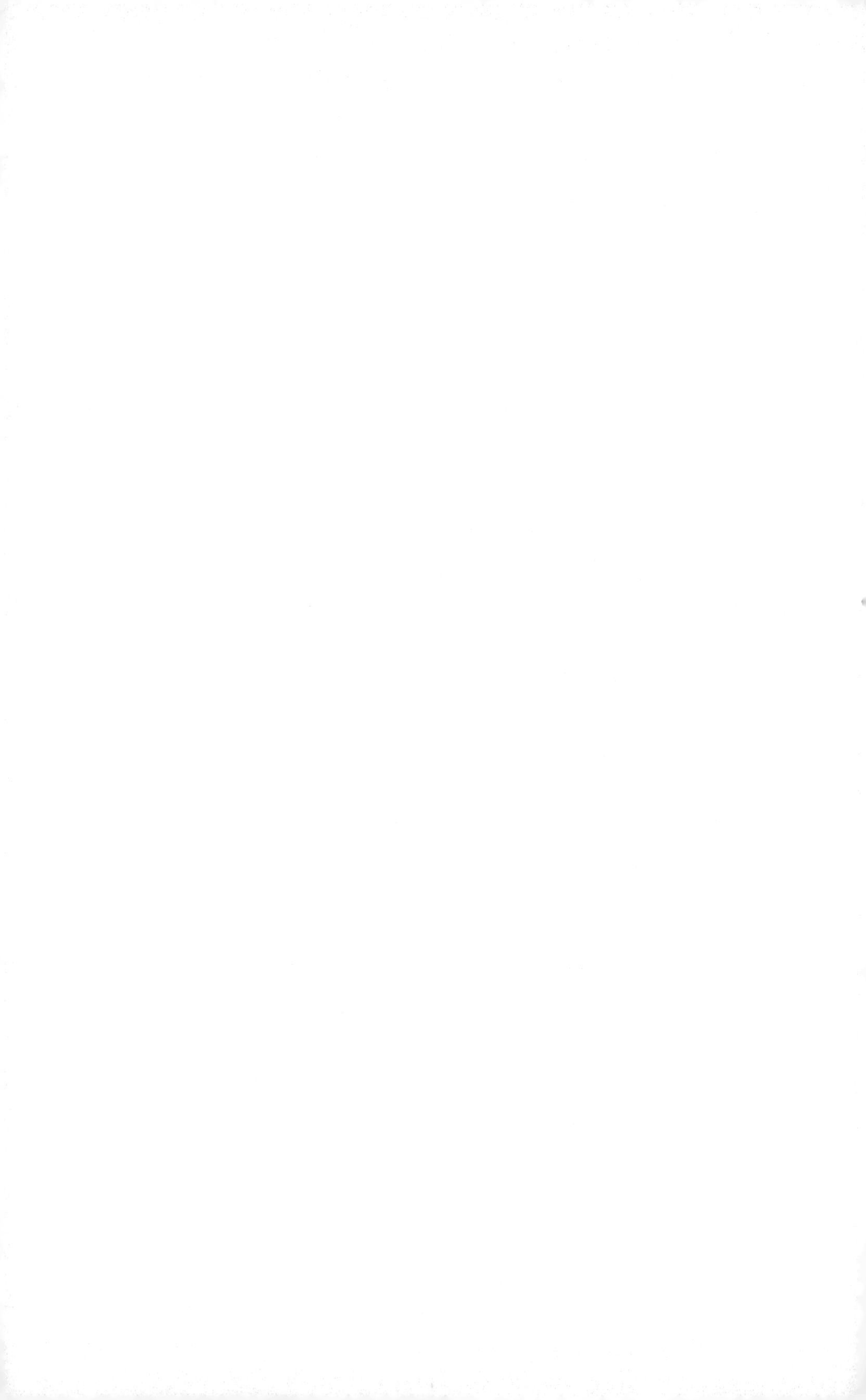

# About the Author

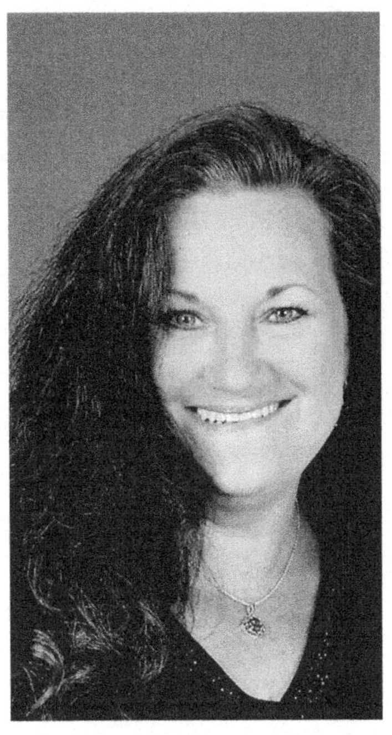

Susan Jeffrey Busen is an award-winning bestselling author, investigative health coach, and international speaker. She helps find solutions for people and animals who are struggling with physical or emotional problems.

She is a former environmental biologist and research scientist whose own health challenges led her to explore natural health, healing, and numerous holistic modalities. She is an avid researcher, an advocate of health freedom, environmental awareness, and is a non-GMO activist. Susan is the founder of GetSet™ Tapping, Tap into Balance, and My Pet Healer.

Susan's passions include helping people overcome life's traumas by releasing negative emotions such as fear, anxiety, and grief, and utilizing her years of expertise in research to educate individuals in private sessions and in group events for schools, hospitals, businesses, and organizations.

Susan believes the body has an incredible wisdom and innate ability to heal itself if given what it needs. Through identifying sensitivities, imbalances, and stressors, she has helped thousands of people optimize their health and excel beyond their limitations. Susan offers remote services to help those who are unable to travel to her.

Visit www.TapintoBalance.com for additional information and resources.

Susan can be contacted at Susan@TapintoBalance.com

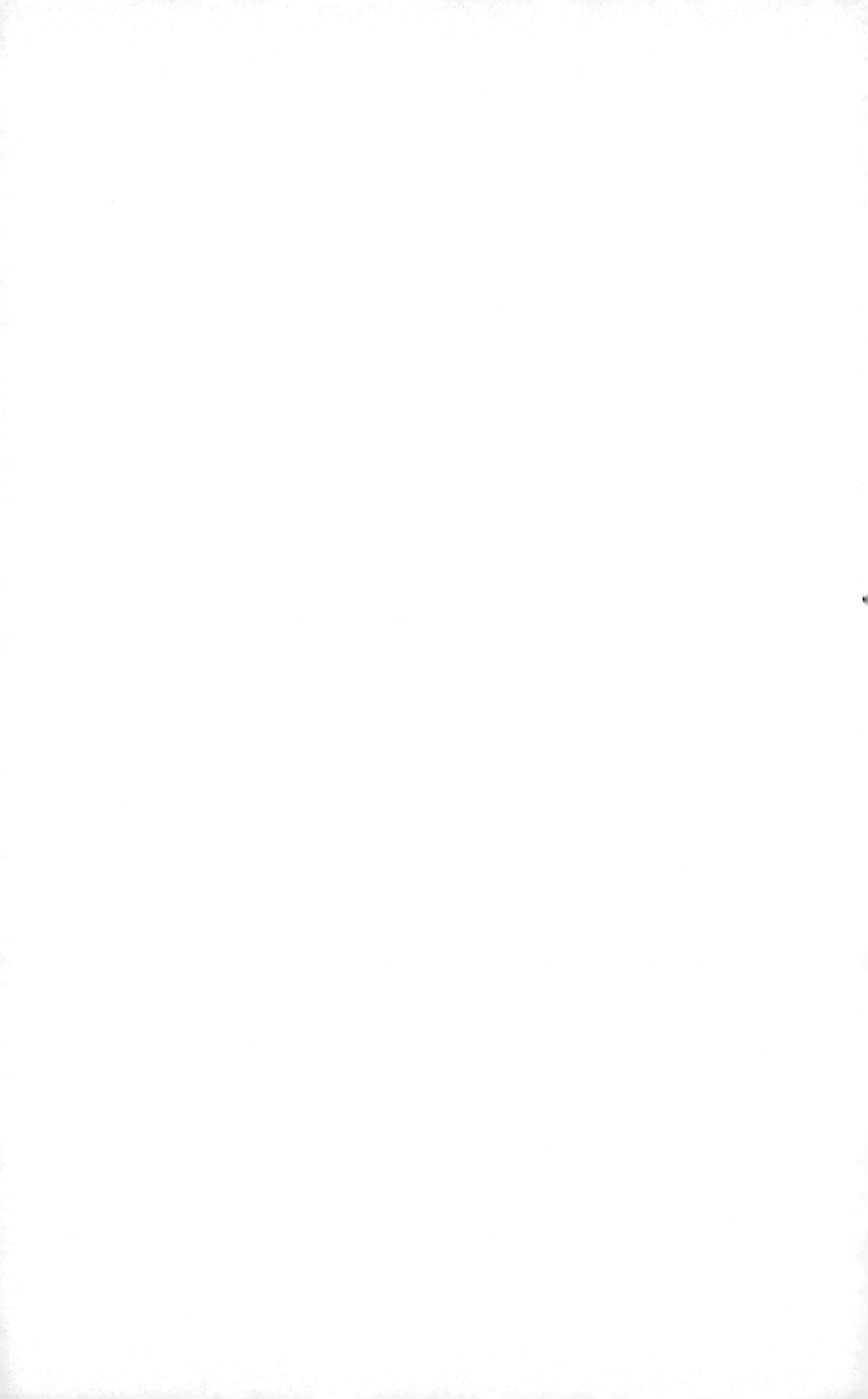

Made in the USA
Monee, IL
10 June 2023

35474912R00174